ADOLESCENT MEDICINE: STATE OF THE ART REVIEWS

Adolescent Contraception: Basics and Beyond

GUEST EDITORS

Paritosh Kaul, MD

Maria Trent, MD, MPH

Krishna K. Upadhya, MD, MPH

Spring 2019 • Volume 30 • Number 1

THE AMERICAN ACADEMY OF PEDIATRICS®

ADOLESCENT MEDICINE:
STATE OF THE ART REVIEWS
Spring 2019
Editor: Carrie Peters
Marketing Manager: Linda Smessaert
Production Manager: Shannan Martin

Volume 30, Number 1
ISBN 978-1-61002-262-0
ISSN 1934-4287
MA0901
SUB1006

The recommendations in this publication do not indicate an exclusive course of treatment or serve as a standard of medical care. Variations, taking into account individual circumstances, may be appropriate.

Statements and opinions expressed are those of the author and not necessarily those of the American Academy of Pediatrics.

Products and Web sites are mentioned for informational purposes only. Inclusion in this publication does not imply endorsement by the American Academy of Pediatrics. The American Academy of Pediatrics is not responsible for the content of the resources mentioned in this publication. Web site addresses are as current as possible but may change at any time.

Every effort has been made to ensure that the drug selection and dosage set forth in this text are in accordance with the current recommendations and practice at the time of publication. It is the responsibility of the health care provider to check the package insert of each drug for any change in indications and dosage and for added warnings and precautions.

Adolescent Medicine: State of the Art Reviews is published 2 times per year by the American Academy of Pediatrics, 345 Park Blvd, Itasca, IL 60143. Periodicals postage paid at Arlington Heights, IL.

POSTMASTER: Send address changes to AM:STARs, American Academy of Pediatrics, Attn: Customer Service Center, 345 Park Blvd, Itasca, IL 60143.

Back issues of *Adolescent Medicine: State of the Art Reviews* (AM:STARs) are available; please visit **shop.aap.org** for more information.

Disclosures: Dr Berlan reports being a certified Nexplanon trainer (Merck). Dr Hoopes reports a Bayer/North American Young Investigator Award. Dr Yen indicates a stock ownership relationship with Pandia Health.

Adolescent Medicine: State of the Art Reviews

Official Journal of the American Academy of Pediatrics
Section on Adolescent Health

ADOLESCENT CONTRACEPTION: BASICS AND BEYOND

EDITOR IN CHIEF

VICTOR C. STRASBURGER, MD, Distinguished Professor Emeritus of Pediatrics, Founding Chief, Division of Adolescent Medicine, University of New Mexico, School of Medicine, Bennington, Vermont

GUEST EDITORS

PARITOSH KAUL, MD, Professor of Pediatrics, Section of Adolescent Medicine, University of Colorado School of Medicine, Children's Hospital Colorado, Aurora, Colorado

MARIA TRENT, MD, MPH, Professor of Pediatrics, Section of Adolescent Medicine, Johns Hopkins University School of Medicine, Johns Hopkins Children's Center, Baltimore, Maryland

KRISHNA K. UPADHYA, MD, MPH, Assistant Professor, Division of Adolescent and Young Adult Medicine, Children's National Health System, Washington, DC

CONTRIBUTORS

ELIZABETH ALDERMAN, MD, Professor of Pediatrics, Department of Pediatrics, Division of Adolescent Medicine, Children's Hospital at Montefiore, Bronx, New York

DAVID L. BELL, MD, MPH, Department of Pediatrics, Columbia University College of Physicians and Surgeons, New York, New York, New York Presbyterian Hospital, New York, New York, Heilbrunn Department of Population and Family Health, Columbia University Mailman School of Public Health, New York, New York

ELISE BERLAN, MD, MPH, Associate Professor of Pediatrics, The Ohio State University College of Medicine, Division of Adolescent Medicine, Nationwide Children's Hospital, Columbus Ohio

ANDREA E. BONNY, MD, Associate Professor of Pediatrics, The Ohio State University College of Medicine, Columbus, Ohio, Research Director, Division of Adolescent Medicine, Nationwide Children's Hospital, Columbus, Ohio

ERICA P. CAHILL, MD, Department of Obstetrics and Gynecology, Stanford Medical School, Palo Alto, California

SUSAN M. COUPEY, MD, Professor of Pediatrics, Chief Emerita, Division of Adolescent Medicine, Children's Hospital at Montefiore, Albert Einstein College of Medicine, Bronx, New York

CASEY COTTRILL, MD, MPH, Assistant Professor of Pediatrics, The Ohio State University College of Medicine, Division of Adolescent Medicine, Nationwide Children's Hospital, Columbus, Ohio

KATHRYN M. CURTIS, PhD, Division of Reproductive Health, Centers for Disease Control and Prevention, Atlanta, Georgia

SHAMIEKA VIRELLA DIXON, MD, Atrium Health's Levine Children's Hospital, Teen Health Connection, Assistant Professor of Pediatrics, Charlotte, North Carolina

J. DENNIS FORTENBERRY, MD, MS, Department of Pediatrics, Division of Adolescent Medicine, Indiana University School of Medicine, Indianapolis, Indiana

KATHRYN GANNON-LOEW, MD, MS, Adolescent Medicine Fellow, Nationwide Children's Hospital, Columbus, Ohio

MELANIE A. GOLD, DO, DMQ, Professor of Pediatrics, Columbia University Irving Medical Center, Professor of Population and Family Health, Mailman School of Public Health, Medical Director, School Based Health Centers, New York-Presbyterian Hospital, New York, New York

LAURA K. GRUBB, MD, MPH, Director, Adolescent Medicine, Assistant Professor of Pediatrics, Assistant Professor of Public Health and Community Medicine, Floating Hospital for Children at Tufts Medical Center, Boston, Massachusetts

ALEXIS GUZMAN, MD, Department of Pediatrics, Columbia University College of Physicians and Surgeons, New York, New York, New York Presbyterian Hospital, New York, New York

ANDREA J. HOOPES, MD, MPH, Adolescent Center, Washington Permanente Medical Group, Seattle, Washington

MEGAN JACOBS, MD, Assistant Professor of Pediatrics, Adolescent Health and Medicine, Oregon Health and Science University, Doernbecher Children's Hospital, Portland, Oregon

TARA C. JATLAOUI, MD, MPH, Division of Reproductive Health, Centers for Disease Control and Prevention, Atlanta, Georgia

PARITOSH KAUL, MD, Professor of Pediatrics, Section of Adolescent Medicine, University of Colorado School of Medicine, Children's Hospital Colorado, Aurora, Colorado

HANNAH L.H. LANGE, MPH, Clinical Research Team Lead, Division of Adolescent Medicine, Nationwide Children's Hospital, Columbus, Ohio

SOFYA MASLYANSKAYA, MD, Assistant Professor of Pediatrics, Division of Adolescent Medicine, Children's Hospital at Montefiore, Albert Einstein College of Medicine, Bronx, New York

SAMUEL O. MASTER, DO, Section of Adolescent Medicine, Department of Pediatrics, Columbia University Irving Medical Center, New York-Presbyterian Hospital, New York, New York

GINA S. SUCATO, MD, MPH, Director, Adolescent Center, Washington Permanente Medical Group, Adjunct Investigator, Kaiser Permanente Washington Health Research Institute, Seattle, Washington

ORQUIDIA TORRES, MD, MS, Assistant Professor of Pediatrics, Department of Pediatrics, Division of Adolescent Medicine, Children's Hospital at Montefiore, Bronx, New York

KRISHNA K. UPADHYA, MD, MPH, Assistant Professor, Division of Adolescent and Young Adult Medicine, Children's National Health System, Washington, DC

SOPHIA YEN, MD, MPH, Division of Adolescent Medicine, Department of Pediatrics, Stanford Medical School, Palo Alto, California

LAUREN B. ZAPATA, PhD, Division of Reproductive Health, Centers for Disease Control and Prevention, Atlanta, Georgia

ADOLESCENT CONTRACEPTION: BASICS AND BEYOND

CONTENTS

Special thanks to Dr Victor Strasburger, who served (with Dr Donald Greydanus) as coeditors in chief for *Adolescent Medicine: State of the Art Reviews* and its prior iterations from 1990 to 2018. We are grateful for his unwavering service to the American Academy of Pediatrics and the Section on Adolescent Health, his commitment to producing a high-quality journal providing continuing education to generations of clinicians, and his continued leadership in the field of Pediatrics and Adolescent Medicine. He is a true warrior for resources to promote the well-being of teens and his work continues to inspire the next generation of pediatricians who simultaneously see both the vulnerability and greatness of young people. We look forward to his ongoing involvement in the Section, his support for the transition of important adolescent content to a new format and wish him continued success in his future endeavors.

Maria Trent, MD, MPH, FSAHM, FAAP
Chair, AAP Section on Adolescent Health

Adolesc Med 030 (2019) xv–xvi

Preface

Adolescent Contraception: Basics and Beyond

Adolescent Medicine: State of the Art Reviews (AM:STARs) has provided state-of-the-art updates for clinicians in the field of adolescent health for the last 25 years. This has been under the stewardship of the coeditors in chief Drs Victor Strasburger and Donald Greydanus, and this issue is no exception. We are especially grateful for the hard work and contributions of each of the authors who provided manuscripts to this issue, which will mark the end of an era of scholarship for our field.

Contraceptive care for adolescents in the current environment challenges pediatricians to stay abreast of an evolving evidence base for methods and counseling, contemplate acquiring new procedural skills, implement new practice models, and navigate a changing policy landscape. The articles in this issue address this range of needs by providing fresh perspectives on contraception in light of the current range of available methods, patient preferences, and innovations in availability. Articles specifically address what clinicians need to know about the benefits and adverse effects of these methods, guidelines for management of commonly encountered adverse effects, and practical advice for incorporating delivery of implants and intrauterine devices into a practice. Finally, although youth today have a variety of contraceptive options, no single method is ideal for every patient. This issue includes articles that focus on novel cases and new contraceptive methods that are on the horizon.

Apart from the content of each article, this issue has 2 additional features. Each article has learning objectives and multiple-choice questions (MCQ). Educational literature supports this approach to acquiring and retaining knowledge. Although the MCQs do not have any continuing medical education credit, they could serve as a review strategy for our readers or as education for all learners in adolescent health.

We would like to acknowledge the support we have received from Carrie Peters, the managing editor of *AM:STARs*. Thank you for your willingness to share your expertise with us. We are writing this preface because of our mentors, patients, and families: they are the fuel that keeps our engine moving. To each other, we are grateful for the opportunity to work together, to learn from each other, and to inspire each other in ways that enhanced our professional and personal growth leading to a better issue of *AM:STARs*.

Paritosh Kaul, MD
Maria Trent, MD, MPH
Krishna K. Upadhya, MD, MPH

Adolesc Med 030 (2019) 1–9

Contraceptive Use by US Adolescents: Where Are We Now?

Krishna K. Upadhya, MD, MPH

Assistant Professor, Division of Adolescent and Young Adult Medicine, Children's National Health System, Washington, DC

LEARNING OBJECTIVES

After reviewing this article, the reader should be able to:

1. Be familiar with the epidemiology of sexual activity and contraceptive use among adolescents in the United States
2. Identify the full range of contraceptive options, both hormonal and non-hormonal, that are available for use by adolescents in the United States
3. Appreciate that variations in sexual activity, contraceptive use, and birth-rates exist across populations as a result of factors including economics, relationship contexts, historical experiences with fertility control, and cultural beliefs
4. Recognize the role of pediatricians in assisting adolescents to overcome barriers to contraceptive access to achieve optimal sexual and reproductive health outcomes

Contraception refers to any method used to prevent pregnancy. Contraception is an important tool that enables adolescents (and adults) to reduce the risk of unwanted pregnancy associated with vaginal intercourse. Because adolescence is a time when many youth begin developing romantic relationships and exploring sexual activity, pediatricians have an important role in ensuring adolescents are able to access contraception to reduce the likelihood of unintended pregnancy. It is also important for pediatricians and other primary care clinicians to provide anticipatory guidance about contraception regardless of an adolescent's immediate needs. Although the average age of first intercourse has remained stable at approximately 17 years,[1] the average age of women at first birth has been increasing in the United States (US), most recently reported at just under

E-mail address: kupadhya@childrensnational.org

 ISSN 1934-4287

27 years.[2] Given the large gap in years between onset of sex and first birth, it makes sense that 99% of US women of reproductive age who have had vaginal intercourse have used contraception.[3] In addition to preventing pregnancy, many available methods of contraception provide benefits such as reducing the pain and bleeding associated with menses, which can improve quality of life and reduce morbidity.

The National Survey of Family Growth, a nationally representative sample of reproductive-age persons (15-49 years) in the United States, indicates that 42% of female and 44% of male 15 to 19 years old have a history of vaginal sexual intercourse with an opposite sex partner. The likelihood of intercourse increases significantly across adolescence, from 11% of females and 15% of males at age 15 to 55% of males and females by age 18, when the rate is not statistically significantly different for males and females.[4] The most recent Youth Risk Behavior Surveillance System survey from 2017, which reflects a representative sample of high school students, indicates that 39.5% of students report a history of sexual intercourse.[5] This percentage has been decreasing over the last 2 cycles. The Youth Risk Behavior Surveillance System has also begun collecting more information about sexual identity reported by students. In the 2017 survey, 85.4% of students identified as heterosexual, 2.4% as gay or lesbian, 8.0% as bisexual, and 4.2% as not sure.[5] Additionally, 45.3% of students had sexual contact with only the opposite sex, 1.6% with only the same sex, and 5.3% with both sexes.[5]

Today's youth have many more contraceptive options available to them than any previous generation. These methods will be detailed in other articles in this issue of AM:STARs. There is now broad consensus among clinical societies, including the American Academy of Pediatrics (AAP), Society for Adolescent Health and Medicine (SAHM), and American College of Obstetricians and Gynecologists (ACOG), that adolescents, regardless of parity, should be considered candidates for an intrauterine device (IUD). Currently 4 hormonal IUDs plus the copper IUD are marketed in the United States, and all have typical use failure rates under 1%.[6] Youth also are candidates for the progestin-only contraceptive implant, which provides up to 3 years of contraception and has a failure rate of approximately 0.05%.[6] In addition to these more recent technologies, the progestin injectable, combined and progestin-only pills, and combined hormonal patch and ring provide significant protection from pregnancy as well as noncontraceptive benefits related to reduced menstrual bleeding.

Non-hormonal contraceptive options remain highly popular among youth, which may reflect ongoing barriers to accessing clinical reproductive health services. Condoms, which provide less effective pregnancy protection compared to hormonal and intrauterine methods (typical use failure rate of 18% for male condoms and 21% for female condoms[6]), uniquely protect against sexually transmitted infections (STIs) and remain the most commonly used method among US adolescents.[4] Importantly, many youth continue to rely on withdrawal, a method that has a typical use failure rate of 22%[6] and provides no protection from STIs. Finally, fertility awareness-based approaches to pregnancy prevention are preferred by some for religious reasons because they do not involve hormones. The effectiveness of these methods among adolescents whose menstrual patterns are still developing is of concern, and they are not generally recommended in clinical guidelines.

As of the most recent report from the Centers for Disease Control and Prevention (CDC) National Survey of Family Growth, nearly 100% of 15- to 19-year-olds who have had vaginal intercourse reported that they used some method of contraception.[4] This high level is driven largely by the use of condoms (Figure 1). In spite of national guidelines recommending implants and IUDs, these devices are used by only a small proportion of youth. Based on the last the last 2 CDC reports, ever use of the implant among 15- to 19-year-olds increased from 1% to 3%; however, there was no statistically significant increase in report of ever use of IUDs (3%).[4] It should also be noted that approximately 20% of teens use no method of contraception at first sex, and use of hormonal or intrauterine (highly effective) methods of contraception is particularly low.[4] Pediatric clinicians are

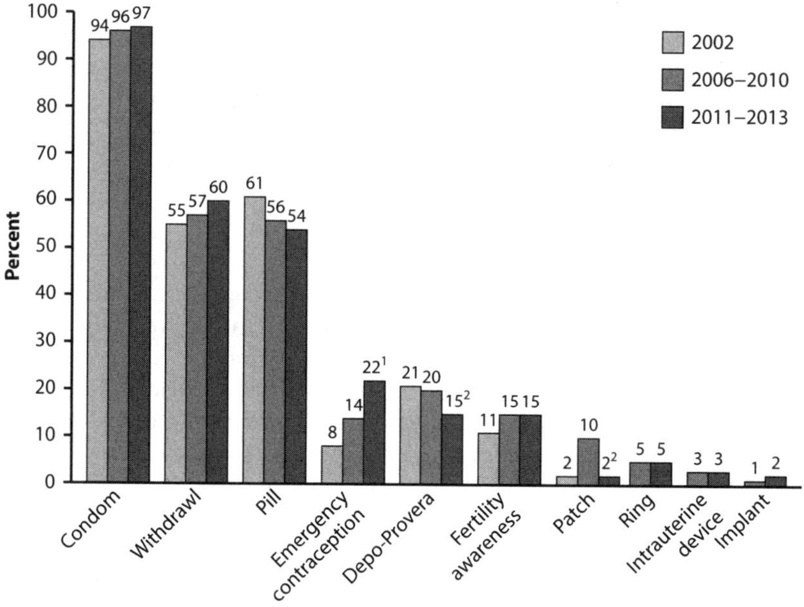

[1] The percentage of female teenagers who ever used emergency contraception increased in 2006–2010 and in 2011–2013 ($p < 0.05$).

[2] Difference in percentage of female teenagers who ever used Depo-Provera or the patch was significantly lower in 2011–2013 than in 2006–2010 ($p < 0.05$).

NOTES: Neither the contraceptive ring nor the implant were available in 2002. The number of teenagers who had ever used the IUD in 2002 was too small to be statistically reliable.

SOURCE: CDC/NCHS, National Survey of Family Growth, 2002, 2006–2010, and 2011–2013.

Fig 1. Methods of contraception ever used among females aged 15-19 who had ever had sexual intercourse: United States, 2002, 2006-2010, 2011-2013.

ideally suited to improve rates of contraceptive use at first sex by offering anticipatory guidance and providing highly effective contraceptive methods beginning early in adolescence.

The high rate of contraceptive use has contributed significantly to the declining rates of teens becoming pregnant and giving birth in the United States over the past several decades. The teen birthrate reached an all-time low in 2016.[7] Importantly, regional and demographic variations in teen births persist.[8] One reason for this is differential access to contraception. Adolescents may be particularly affected by barriers to access, including reluctance to seek contraceptive care due to stigma surrounding teen sexual behavior, lack of confidentiality because of coverage under parents' insurance policies,[9,10] limited independent financial resources, and state restrictions on ability to consent for services.[11] Publicly funded family planning clinics (most notably those funded under the federal grant program Title X) have been an important resource for adolescents seeking low-cost and confidential access to services.[12] Title X clinics have been shown to be more likely than other clinic types to offer high-quality care and a full range of contraceptive options.[12] Unfortunately, these publicly funded clinics are not uniformly available. The National Campaign to Prevent Teen and Unplanned Pregnancy (now known as Power to Decide) collects data on the geographic locations of publicly funded contraceptive clinics, including the presence of "contraceptive deserts," defined as areas where women lack reasonable access to a public clinic with the full range of methods.[13] Policy proposals currently under consideration that would restrict Title X family planning funding from sites that refer to or provide abortion services could further reduce clinic numbers and could have a disproportionate negative effect on adolescents. A state implementation of this policy in Texas resulted in reduced access to contraception and abortion and increased rates of unwanted pregnancies.[14]

Variations and disparities in rates of teen birth among communities are also driven by other individual and social determinants. Studies over many decades have shown associations between neighborhood economic factors and likelihood of teen birth.[15] Other data support that relationship context and an individual's perception of risk for STI also influence contraceptive use.[16,17] Religious and cultural beliefs along with historical experiences with fertility control in some minority groups are other key factors influencing the use of contraception and teen fertility.

Any discussion of contraception and trends in contraceptive use must include an acknowledgment of the fact that the reproduction of certain populations is often valued more than that of other populations in a society. This has led to policy proposals that dictate or incentivize use of contraceptive methods by poor and minority women and selective marketing of certain contraceptive methods. Examples of these policies include those authorizing sterilization of poor women without their consent and making public benefits contingent on use of Norplant during the 1990s.[18] It is important that pediatricians and other clinicians are aware of this history and consider its effect on contemporary reproductive health discussions. In order to ensure the most patient-centered approach to contraceptive counseling, starting from the perspective of reproductive justice can be instructive. As defined by Hoopes and Sucato in an article on intrauterine devices in this issue of AM:STARs, a reproductive justice framework is "one that upholds the human right to maintain personal bodily autonomy, have children, not have children, and parent children in safe and sustainable communities." This approach was explicitly advocated by ACOG in their most recent Committee Opinion on Adolescent Pregnancy, Contraception and Sexual Activity.[19]

Along with the range of available methods, clinicians today have an abundance of guidelines and resources to help implement high-quality, evidence-based contraceptive care in their practices. As reviewed in depth in an article on adolescent pregnancy prevention by Zapata et al. in this issue of AM:STARs, the CDC has published the U.S. Medical Eligibility Criteria for Contraceptive Use, which clinicians can consult to determine whether a particular contraceptive method is contraindicated based on a medical condition.[20] Information on starting or discontinuing methods, timing of backup methods, and management of common adverse effects are outlined in the CDC's US Selected Practice Recommendations for Contraceptive Use.[21] Additional federal guidance on providing high-quality contraceptive care is available in the Update: Providing Quality Family Planning Services—Recommendations from CDC and the US Office of Population Affairs.[22] The American Academy of Pediatrics policy statement on contraception also provides guidance for pediatricians.[23] Finally, guidance for clinicians[24] on how to make a reproductive health visit most "adolescent friendly" is available (Figure 2).[24]

Despite the relatively wide range of methods available to today's youth, no available method is perfect, and allaying fear of or minimizing unwanted adverse effects is critical to contraceptive uptake and continuation. It is important that pediatric clinicians are honest with their patients about these adverse effects and open to the fact that they may outweigh any potential benefits when viewed from the patient's perspective. Clinicians also need to recognize that unwanted pregnancy is not the only threat to optimal sexual and reproductive health facing youth. The CDC data indicate that adolescents and young adults account for half of all STI diagnoses in the United States despite making up only one-fourth of the sexually active population.[25] The CDC also reports that the rates of chlamydia, gonorrhea, and syphilis infection among adolescents and young adults increased between 2012 and 2016.[25] As is the case with teen births, the rates of these infections, as well as that of human immunodeficiency virus, are not equally distributed across the country.[26] Youth in communities with the highest rates of infection face multiple challenges to their reproductive futures. Pediatricians are ideally situated to help youth identify and manage these challenges and

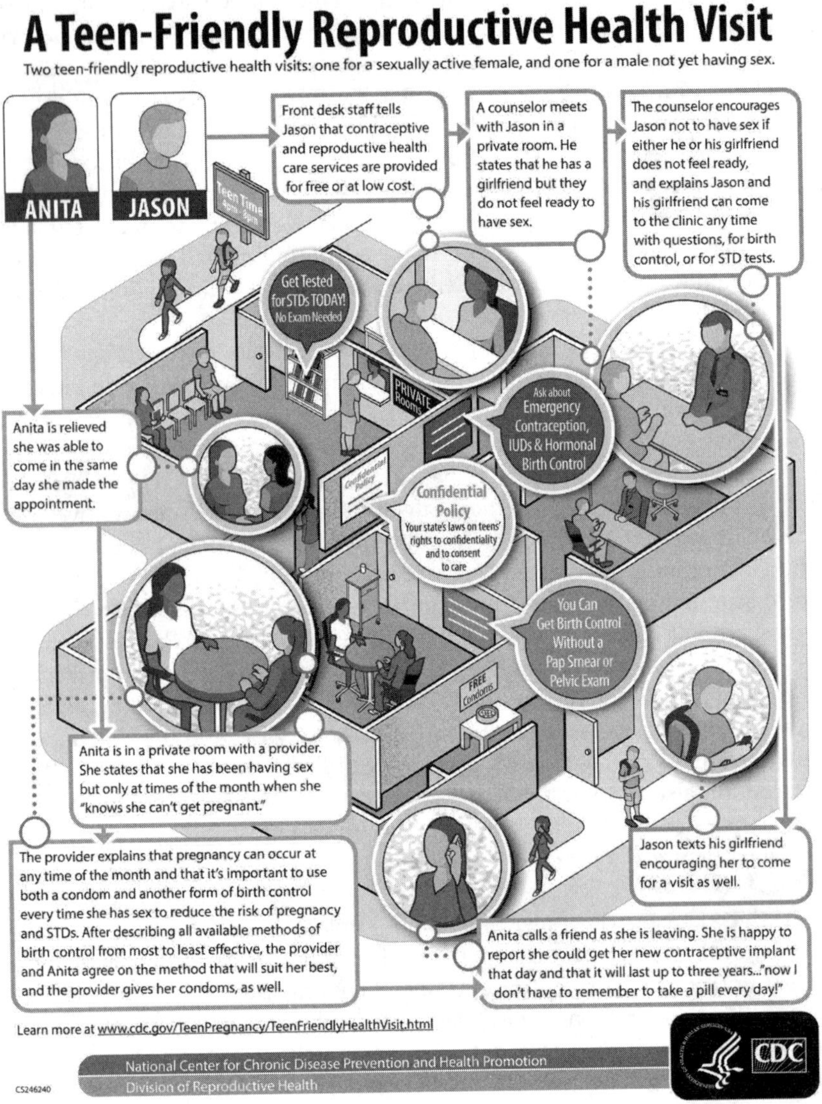

Fig 2. Infographic highlighting important aspects of a teen friendly reproductive health visit. Centers for Disease Control and Prevention. Infographic: teen-friendly reproductive health visit. https://www.cdc.gov/teenpregnancy/health-care-providers/teen-friendly-health-visit.htm. Updated September 5, 2013. Accessed August 28, 2018.

to educate the public about their unique needs. As outlined in an article on policy foundations supporting adolescent access to contraceptive care by Grubb and Upadhya in this issue of AM:STARs, policies and programs that support affordable and confidential access to contraception and other reproductive health services, notably Medicaid and Title X, are an important backbone supporting adolescents, and many opportunities exist for pediatricians to advocate for the continuation and strengthening of these policies and programs.

In summary, the contraceptive options we can offer in pediatric and adolescent medicine today are greater than ever, but we must remain vigilant to ensure that all youth can benefit from the advances to date. In addition, we must continue to work to develop better technologies and implementation approaches for the future.

QUESTIONS

1. Over the past decade, the consensus of medical organizations has shifted to endorse use of intrauterine devices (IUDs) in adolescents regardless of parity. Data indicate that since then:
   A. Use of IUDs by US teens has increased and use of condoms has remained stable.
   B. Use of IUDs by US teens has not changed and use of condoms has remained stable.
   C. Use of IUDs by US teens has not changed and use of condoms has increased.
   D. Use of IUDs by US teens has increased and use of condoms has decreased.
2. Data on sexual activity and contraceptive use are important to collect in order to identify trends and areas for intervention. In the United States, 2 critical sources of data on youth include:
   A. The Youth Risk Behavior Surveillance System conducted biannually to produce a nationally representative sample of high school students and the National Survey of Family Growth conducted continuously to produce a nationally representative sample of reproductive-age persons (15-49 years).
   B. The Youth Risk Behavior Surveillance System conducted biannually to produce a nationally representative sample of 13- to 18-year-olds and the National Survey of Family Growth conducted continuously to produce a nationally representative sample of reproductive-age persons (15-44 years).
   C. The Youth Risk Behavior Surveillance System conducted annually to produce a nationally representative sample of 13- to 18-year-olds and the National Survey of Family Growth conducted continuously to produce a nationally representative sample of reproductive-age persons (12-44 years).

D. The Youth Risk Behavior Surveillance System conducted biannually to produce a nationally representative sample of high school students and the National Survey of Family Growth conducted continuously to produce a nationally representative sample of reproductive-age persons (12-44 years).

3. In order to facilitate an adolescent's selection of an appropriate contraceptive method, the best approach for pediatricians is to:
   A. Provide tiered effectiveness counseling, starting with the most effective and moving to the least effective methods because risk of failure is the determining factor for most teens.
   B. Refer to a reproductive health specialist who can provide comprehensive counseling about all methods and place IUDs.
   C. Provide comprehensive counseling about all available methods, including implants and IUDs, with tailoring to the factors identified as most important to the patient.
   D. Elicit medical contraindications before counseling about IUDs because contraindications to their use are common.

(See page 196 for answers.)

References

1. Centers for Disease Control and Prevention. Key statistics from the National Survey of Family Growth–S listing. https://www.cdc.gov/nchs/nsfg/key_statistics/s.htm#vaginalsexual. Updated August 14, 2017. Accessed August 28, 2018
2. Martin JA, Hamilton BE, Osterman MJK, Driscoll AK, Drake P. Births: final data for 2016. National Vital Statistics Reports; vol 67, no 1. Hyattsville, MD: National Center for Health Statistics; 2018
3. Guttmacher Institute. Contraceptive use in the United States. July 2018 Fact Sheet. https://www.guttmacher.org/fact-sheet/contraceptive-use-united-states. Accessed August 28, 2018
4. Abma JC, Martinez GM. Sexual activity and contraceptive use among teenagers in the United States, 2011–2015. *Natl Health Stat Report.* 2017;104:1-23
5. Kann L, McManus T, Harris WA, et al. Youth Risk Behavior Surveillance—United States, 2017. *MMWR Surveill Summ.* 2018;67(8):1-479
6. Centers for Disease Control and Prevention. Effectiveness of family planning methods. http://www.cdc.gov/reproductivehealth/contraception/unintendedpregnancy/pdf/Contraceptive_methods_508.pdf. Updated August 29, 2013. Accessed August 28, 2018
7. Martin JA, Hamilton BE, Osterman MJK. Births in the United States, 2016. NCHS Data Brief; no 287. Hyattsville, MD: National Center for Health Statistics; 2017
8. Romero L, Pazol K, Warner L, et al. Reduced disparities in birth rates among teens aged 15–19 years—United States, 2006–2007 and 2013–2014. *MMWR Morb Mortal Wkly Rep.* 2016;65: 409-414
9. Copen CE, Dittus PJ, Leichliter JS. Confidentiality concerns and sexual and reproductive health care among adolescents and young adults aged 15–25. NCHS Data Brief; no 266. Hyattsville, MD: National Center for Health Statistics; 2016
10. Fuentes l, Ingerick M, Jones R, Lindberg L. Adolescents' and young adults' reports of barriers to confidential health care and receipt of contraceptive services. *J Adolesc Health.* 2018;62(1):36-43
11. Guttmacher Institute. An overview of minors' consent laws. August 2018. https://www.guttmacher.org/state-policy/explore/overview-minors-consent-law. Updated August 1, 2018. Accessed August 28, 2018

12. Wood SF, Strasser J, Sharac J, et al. Community health centers and family planning in an era of policy uncertainty. Kaiser Family Foundation, Washington DC. March 15, 2018. https://www.kff.org/report-section/community-health-centers-and-family-planning-in-an-era-of-policy-uncertainty-report. Accessed August 28, 2018
13. Power to Decide. Access to birth control: lack of access = lack of power to decide. https://powertodecide.org/what-we-do/access/access-birth-control. Accessed August 28, 2018
14. Stevenson AJ, Flores-Vazquez IM, Allgeyer RL, Schenkkan P, Potter JE. Effect of removal of Planned Parenthood from the Texas Women's Health Program. *N Engl J Med.* 2016;374:853-860
15. Penman-Aguilar A, Carter M, Snead MC, Kourtis AP. Socioeconomic disadvantage as a social determinant of teen childbearing in the U.S. *Public Health Rep.* 2013;128(Suppl 1):5-22
16. Raine T, Minnis AM, Padian NS. Determinants of contraceptive method among young women at risk for unintended pregnancy and sexually transmitted infections. *Contraception.* 2003;68(1):19-25
17. Manlove J, Ryan S, Franzetta K. Contraceptive use patterns across teens' sexual relationships: the role of relationships, partners, and sexual histories. *Demography.* 2007;44(3):603-621
18. Harris LH, Wolfe T. Stratified reproduction, family planning care and the double edge of history. *Curr Opin Obstet Gynecol.* 2014;26:539-544
19. American College of Obstetricians and Gynecologists Committee on Adolescent Health Care. Committee Opinion No. 699: adolescent pregnancy, contraception, and sexual activity. *Obstet Gynecol.* 2017;129:e142-e149
20. Curtis KM, Tepper NK, Jatlaoui TC, et al. U.S. Medical Eligibility Criteria for Contraceptive Use, 2016. *MMWR Recomm Rep.* 2016;65(3):1-103
21. Curtis KM, Jatlaoui TC, Tepper NK, et al. U.S. Selected Practice Recommendations for Contraceptive Use, 2016. *MMWR Recomm Rep.* 2016;65(4):1-66
22. Gavin L, Pazol K, Ahrens K. Update: Providing Quality Family Planning Services—Recommendations From CDC and the U.S. Office of Population Affairs, 2017. *MMWR Morb Mortal Wkly Rep.* 2017;66:1383-1385
23. American Academy of Pediatrics Committee on Adolescence. Contraception for adolescents. *Pediatrics.* 2014;134(4):e1244-e1256
24. Centers for Disease Control and Prevention. Infographic: teen-friendly reproductive health visit. https://www.cdc.gov/teenpregnancy/health-care-providers/teen-friendly-health-visit.htm. Updated September 5, 2013. Accessed August 28, 2018
25. Centers for Disease Control and Prevention. STDs in adolescents and young adults. https://www.cdc.gov/std/stats16/adolescents.htm. Updated September 26, 2017. Accessed August 28, 2018
26. Ocfemia MC, Dunville R, Zhang T, Barrios LC, Oster AM. HIV diagnoses among persons aged 13–29 years—United States, 2010–2014. *MMWR Morb Mortal Wkly Rep.* 2018;67:212-215

Adolesc Med 030 (2019) 10–23

Adolescent Pregnancy Prevention: Application of CDC Evidence-Based Contraception Guidance

Lauren B. Zapata, PhD*; Tara C. Jatlaoui, MD, MPH; Kathryn M. Curtis, PhD

Division of Reproductive Health, Centers for Disease Control and Prevention, Atlanta, Georgia

LEARNING OBJECTIVES

After reviewing this article, the reader should be able to:

1. Describe how to use the U.S. Medical Eligibility Criteria for Contraceptive Use to determine safe use of contraceptive methods for adolescents
2. Describe when adolescents can initiate contraception, how to be reasonably certain an adolescent is not pregnant before starting contraception, and which examinations and tests are necessary before starting contraception
3. Describe emergency contraception options for adolescents

INTRODUCTION

Contraception is an important consideration for sexually active adolescents to prevent pregnancy. Although pregnancy, birth, and abortion rates are declining in the United States for teens age 15 to 19 years and reached historic lows in 2013,[1] the United States still has the highest teen birthrate of any industrialized country.[2] In 2013, there were 448,000 pregnancies among females age 15 to 19 years, for a pregnancy rate of 43 per 1000 women in this age group.[1] Contraception is also important to prevent repeat births among teens, defined as 2 or

---

Disclaimer: The findings and conclusions in this report are those of the authors and do not necessarily represent the official position of the CDC.

*Corresponding author
E-mail address: lzapata@cdc.gov

 ISSN 1934-4287

more live births before the age of 20. Although the proportion of teen births that were repeat births decreased from 2004 to 2015, nearly 1 in 5 teen births in 2015 was a repeat birth.[3]

The decline in adolescent pregnancy in the United States has been largely attributed to improvements in contraceptive use among adolescents.[4] Whereas sexual activity among adolescents did not change from 2007 to 2012 based on data from the National Survey of Family Growth, significant increases in the use of any contraceptive method, multiple methods, and highly effective methods were observed. Some of the most effective reversible methods of contraception, based on rates of pregnancy with typical use, are intrauterine devices (IUDs), implants, depot medroxyprogesterone acetate (DMPA), oral contraceptive pills, contraceptive patches, and vaginal rings; condoms and withdrawal are less effective methods.[5] However, teens more often use less effective methods. Among female teenagers 15 to 19 years who had ever had sexual intercourse, 97% had used a condom at least once, 60% had ever used withdrawal, 54% had ever used the pill, and 5% had ever used an IUD or implant.[6]

The objective of this article is to provide an overview of the Centers for Disease Control and Prevention (CDC) evidence-based contraception guidelines that health care professionals can use to remove unnecessary barriers and increase access to safe and effective contraception for adolescents.

CDC EVIDENCE-BASED CONTRACEPTION GUIDANCE

The CDC publishes the U.S. Medical Eligibility Criteria for Contraceptive Use (US MEC)[7] and the U.S. Selected Practice Recommendations for Contraceptive Use (US SPR),[8] both adapted from global guidance developed by the World Health Organization (WHO).[9,10] The goal of the recommendations is to remove unnecessary medical barriers to accessing and using contraception, thus reducing unintended pregnancies. The recommendations are intended to be sources of clinical guidance for health care professionals when counseling women, men, and couples (including adolescents) about family planning. They are based on rigorous identification and critical appraisal of the scientific evidence and input from experts. To maintain the guidance, in collaboration with WHO, the CDC monitors the literature for new evidence relevant to the recommendations through the WHO/CDC Continuous Identification of Research Evidence system.[11]

The US MEC provides evidence-based guidance on the safety of contraceptive methods for women with certain characteristics or medical conditions. For example, is it safe for a postpartum woman to use an IUD? The recommendations refer to contraceptive methods being used for contraceptive purposes and do not consider the use of contraceptive methods for treatment of medical conditions, because the eligibility in these situations might be different. Although

Table 1
US MEC categories

Category	Description
1	A condition for which there is no restriction for the use of the contraceptive method
2	A condition for which the advantages of using the method generally outweigh the theoretical or proven risks
3	A condition for which the theoretical or proven risks usually outweigh the advantages of using the method
4	A condition that represents an unacceptable health risk if the contraceptive method is used

US MEC, U.S. Medical Eligibility Criteria for Contraceptive Use.

the recommendations are intended to be a source of clinical guidance, practitioners should always consider individual clinical circumstances when counseling patients. For each medical condition and personal characteristic included in the US MEC, recommendations are provided using a numeric scheme ranging from category 1 (the method is safe to use without restriction) to category 4 (the method poses an unacceptable health risk) (Table 1). Category 2 indicates that the advantages of using the method generally outweigh any risks, and the method generally can be used. Category 3 requires careful clinical judgment; use of the method is generally not recommended unless other methods are not available or acceptable. The US MEC provides guidance for 17 contraceptive methods and more than 120 medical conditions and personal characteristics.

When considering age as a characteristic, all methods of contraception are considered safe or generally safe for adolescents (category 1 or 2). For the implant, progestin-only pills, and barriers methods, the recommendations are the same for women of all ages (category 1). For combined hormonal contraceptives (CHCs), the methods are classified as category 1 for women age younger than 40 years and category 2 for women age 40 years or older. Intrauterine devices are classified as category 2 for women from menarche up to 20 years and category 1 for women age 20 years or older. Although safe to use, IUDs for younger women receive a category 2 (benefits outweigh risks) for IUDs because of concerns about the somewhat higher risk for expulsion with nulliparity and increased risk for sexually transmitted infections (STIs) from sexual behavior in younger age groups.[7] Depot medroxyprogesterone acetate is classified as category 2 for women from menarche up to 18 years and for women older than 45 years, and category 1 for women age 18 to 45 years. Although studies have found that users of DMPA lose bone mass density during its use and recover bone mineral density after discontinuation, there is concern that some adolescents may not reach their peak bone mass and that perimenopausal women may not fully recover before menopause.[7] Although all methods of contraception are considered safe for adolescents based on their age alone, there may be additional considerations for adolescents with medical conditions or other characteristics. Table 2 summarizes medical conditions and characteristics for which adolescents can safely use a method (category 1 or 2) and situations for which a method may be considered unsafe (category 3 or 4). The full US MEC provides further explanation and recommendations for additional medical conditions.

Table 2
Safety of contraceptive methods for adolescents with select medical conditions or characteristics[a]

Medical condition or characteristic	**IUD**	**Implant**	**DMPA**	**CHC**
Nulliparous	Safe[b]	Safe	Safe	Safe
Postpartum <21 days	Safe	Safe	Safe	Unsafe[c]
Obesity	Safe	Safe	Safe	Safe
History of bariatric surgery via malabsorptive procedures	Safe	Safe	Safe	COCs less effective[d] (category 3) Patch/ring safe
Smoking	Safe	Safe	Safe	Safe
Antimicrobial therapy with broad-spectrum antibiotics, antifungals, or antiparasitics	Safe	Safe	Safe	Safe
Migraine with aura	Safe	Safe	Safe	Unsafe
Migraine without aura	Safe	Safe	Safe	Safe
Depressive disorders	Safe	Safe	Safe	Safe
Family history of breast cancer	Safe	Safe	Safe	Safe
Benign ovarian tumors	Safe	Safe	Safe	Safe
Sickle cell disease	Safe	Safe	Safe	Safe
Cystic fibrosis	Safe	Safe	Safe	Safe
Insulin or non–insulin-dependent diabetes with nonvascular disease	Safe	Safe	Safe	Safe
Past history of pelvic inflammatory disease	Safe	Safe	Safe	Safe
Current pelvic inflammatory disease	Unsafe for initiation Safe for continuation	Safe	Safe	Safe
Current purulent cervicitis or chlamydial infection or gonococcal infection	Unsafe for initiation Safe for continuation	Safe	Safe	Safe
Vaginitis	Safe	Safe	Safe	Safe

CHC, combined hormonal contraceptive; COC, combined oral contraceptive; DMPA, depot medroxyprogesterone acetate; IUD, intrauterine device.

[a] Complete recommendations are listed in the U.S. Medical Eligibility Criteria for Contraceptive Use (US MEC), 2016. https://www.cdc.gov/reproductivehealth/contraception/contraception_guidance.htm.

[b] Safe = US MEC category 1 or 2.

[c] Unsafe = US MEC category 4.

[d] Progestin-only pills (POPs) are also less effective (category 3) for those with history of bariatric surgery via malabsorptive procedures. For complete recommendations for POPs, see the US MEC.

The US SPR is a companion document to the US MEC that addresses a select group of common, yet complex, issues regarding initiation and use of specific contraceptive methods. The US SPR includes topics such as when to start using specific contraceptive methods, how to be reasonably certain that a woman is not pregnant before starting a method, examinations and tests needed before initiation of contraceptive methods, routine follow-up after contraceptive initiation, and management of women with bleeding irregularities and other problems while using contraception. The US SPR also includes recommended actions for women in the event of late DMPA reinjections, late or missed doses of CHCs, and missed progestin-only pills. The recommendations apply to females of all ages, including adolescents. The goal of the US SPR is to reduce barriers to contraception use by providing guidance for how females, including adolescents, can initiate methods easily and continue use effectively. Adolescents, in particular, may face certain barriers to initiating and using contraception effectively, including unnecessary medical examinations, challenges in accessing supplies, and difficulties with adherence. For each recommendation, the US SPR includes simplified text of the recommendation itself, followed by comments and an evidence summary.

To disseminate and promote use of the US MEC and US SPR, several provider tools have been developed and are available on CDC's Division of Reproductive Health website at no cost for download or order (Table 3).

CLINICAL CASE SCENARIOS USING THE US MEC AND US SPR

When a patient presents desiring or using contraception, the US MEC can help guide discussions regarding safety for adolescents with certain characteristics or conditions. Once a patient decides to initiate a particular method or is already using a method, the US SPR guidance can be used to address certain clinical considerations.

Clinical Scenario 1

A 16-year-old nulliparous, healthy female presents to your office. She is currently using condoms with her boyfriend, but she wishes to use a more reliable method and wants to know from which options she can choose.

Although many factors are involved in the choice of a method, safety is an important consideration, and the US MEC provides evidence-based recommendations to guide discussions in selecting a method. For adolescents, all methods, including IUDs and DMPA, are safe options.

Various myths and misperceptions regarding IUD use in adolescents remain. Some practitioners may be concerned about an increased risk for expulsion, which has been shown in some studies; thus, the recommendation for IUD use

Table 3
US MEC and US SPR provider tools[a]

Provider tool	Description
US MEC/US SPR application[a,b]	An easy-to-use reference that combines information from the US MEC and US SPR and features a streamlined interface so providers can access the guidance quickly and easily (available for iOS and Android operating systems)
US MEC/US SPR eBooks[a,b]	Electronic versions of the full guidance documents that can be easily read and searched on electronic devices, including handheld devices
US MEC wheel[a]	An easy-to-use tool similar to a pregnancy gestation wheel that summarizes US MEC classifications; the medical conditions and personal characteristics are around the outside of the wheel, the contraceptive methods around the inside of the wheel, and the recommendations are revealed as the wheel turns
US MEC summary chart[a]	A color-coded summary chart of US MEC classifications for IUDs, implants, DMPA, POPs, and CHCs
US SPR charts[b]	Summary charts (front and back) on the following topics: (1) Front: When to start using specific contraceptive methods (including how to be reasonably certain that a woman is not pregnant) Back: Routine follow-up after contraceptive initiation (2) Front: Recommended actions after late or missed combined oral contraceptives Back: Recommended actions after delayed application or detachment with combined hormonal patch and recommended action after delayed insertion or reinsertion with combined vaginal ring (3) Front: Management of women with bleeding irregularities while using contraception Back: Management of the IUD when an IUD user is found to have pelvic inflammatory disease
US MEC/US SPR speaker-ready slide sets[a,b]	Slide presentations that can be used by providers who want to increase their knowledge about the US MEC/US SPR. The presentations and speaker notes can also be used or adapted to give presentations. Continuing education credits are available

CHC, combined hormonal contraceptive; DMPA, depot medroxyprogesterone acetate; IUD, intrauterine device; POP, progestin-only pill; US MEC, U.S. Medical Eligibility Criteria for Contraceptive Use; US SPR, U.S. Selected Practice Recommendations for Contraceptive Use.
[a] https://www.cdc.gov/reproductivehealth/contraception/mmwr/mec/summary.html.
[b] https://www.cdc.gov/reproductivehealth/contraception/mmwr/spr/summary.html.

in women younger than 20 years is a category 2. They also may be concerned about future fertility, although there is no evidence that IUDs cause later infertility.[12,13] Instead, risk of infertility is associated with gonorrheal and chlamydial infections, which are common among young women.[12,13] Women with current purulent cervicitis, current chlamydial or gonococcal infection, or current pelvic inflammatory disease should not start using an IUD (category 4). If an adolescent has not been screened for gonorrhea and chlamydia according to CDC sexually transmitted diseases treatment guidelines,[14] screening may be performed at the time of IUD insertion, and insertion should not be delayed.[8]

Some practitioners may have concerns about DMPA use among adolescents, specifically related to loss of bone mineral density and weight gain. Bone mineral density is lost, in small amounts, during DMPA use in females (including adolescents), but bone mineral density is regained after discontinuation of DMPA.[7] There is no evidence that DMPA use increases fracture risk in adolescents, and how bone mineral density measures are associated with future fractures in adolescents is unclear. Related to weight gain, obese adolescents using DMPA may be more likely to gain weight compared to non-obese users and obese users of other methods.[7] For these reasons, DMPA is classified as a category 2 for adolescents younger than 18 years.

Given the patient's interest in a more reliable method, in addition to an IUD or DMPA the patient can safely use the implant or CHCs. Regardless of method selected by the patient after counseling, condom use for dual protection against pregnancy and STIs should be encouraged. For any other medical conditions or characteristics, the US MEC can be used to provide additional safety recommendations for consideration.

Clinical Scenario 2

An 18-year-old nulliparous, healthy female presents to your office for her well visit. She has discussed contraception with you in the past and wants to start the contraceptive implant as soon as possible.

The US SPR provides recommendations to assist health care professionals. It includes guidance on when to initiate contraceptive methods, how to be reasonably sure that a woman is not pregnant at the time of initiation, and what examinations and tests are needed before starting a method with the goal of reducing unnecessary obstacles to contraception.

Women may face several barriers to starting contraception, including waiting for their next menses or returning for a second visit. Starting the patient on her chosen method at the time she requests the method, also known as "quick start," may reduce such barriers and the time a woman may be at risk for pregnancy. The US SPR provides guidance (for all methods), both within the document and summarized in a user-friendly chart (Table 4), to guide health care professionals on when to start a method and how to counsel patients on the need for backup contraception. Any of the methods can be started at any time if the practitioner is reasonably certain that the woman is not pregnant. For contraceptive methods other than IUDs (including the implant), if the practitioner is uncertain about whether the woman might be pregnant, the benefits of starting the method likely

Table 4
When to start using specific contraceptive methods

Contraceptive method	When to start[a]	Additional contraception needed (ie, backup)	Examinations or tests needed before initiation[b]
Copper-containing IUD	Any time	Not needed	Bimanual examination and cervical inspection[c]
Levonorgestrel-releasing IUD	Any time	If >7 days after menses started, use backup method or abstain for 7 days	Bimanual examination and cervical inspection[c]
Implant	Any time	If >5 days after menses started, use backup method or abstain for 7 days	None
Injectable	Any time	If >7 days after menses started, use backup method or abstain for 7 days	None
Combined hormonal contraceptive	Any time	If >5 days after menses started, use backup method or abstain for 7 days	Blood pressure measurement
Progestin-only pill	Any time	If >5 days after menses started, use backup method or abstain for 2 days	None

[a] When to start if the provider is reasonably certain that the woman is not pregnant.

[b] Weight (body mass index [BMI]) measurement is not needed to determine medical eligibility for any methods of contraception because all methods can be used (U.S. Medical Eligibility Criteria for Contraceptive Use [US MEC] category 1) or generally can be used (US MEC category 2) among obese women. However, measuring weight and calculating BMI (weight [kg]/height[m^2]) at baseline might be helpful for monitoring any changes and counseling women who might be concerned about weight change perceived to be associated with their contraceptive method.

[c] Most women do not require additional screening for sexually transmitted infections (STI) at the time of intrauterine device (IUD) insertion. If a woman with risk factors for STIs has not been screened for gonorrhea and chlamydia according to the Centers for Disease Control and Prevention sexually transmitted diseases treatment guidelines (https://www.cdc.gov/std/tg2015/default.htm), screening can be performed at the time of IUD insertion, and insertion should not be delayed. Women with current purulent cervicitis or chlamydial infection or gonococcal infection should not undergo IUD insertion (US MEC category 4).

From When to Start Using Specific Contraceptive Methods. https://www.cdc.gov/reproductivehealth/contraception/pdf/When-To-Start_508Tagged.pdf. Accessed October 29, 2018.

exceed any risk, and the method can be initiated with a follow-up pregnancy test in 2 to 4 weeks. For IUDs, if the practitioner is uncertain about whether the patient might be pregnant, the woman should be offered another method until the practitioner is reasonably certain that the patient is not pregnant and the IUD can be safely inserted.

The copper (Cu)-IUD begins working immediately, whereas other methods require backup contraception if not initiated at the beginning of a woman's cycle.

In order to prevent pregnancy until hormonal contraceptive methods begin working most effectively, a practitioner needs to discuss backup contraception or abstinence (Table 4). For the implant, if it has been more than 5 days since the woman's last cycle started, she will need to use a backup method or abstain from sexual intercourse for 7 days after the implant has been initiated. For women who may not have a last menstrual cycle to use as a reference to (eg, women who are amenorrheic, postpartum, postabortion, or switching from another method), the US SPR includes guidance on initiation in these situations; the recommendations can be found under each contraceptive method in the "Initiation" section.

Some practitioners may question whether they should order a pregnancy test to rule out pregnancy and whether the result of a pregnancy test is accurate. Pregnancy testing has limitations, with pregnancy detection rates varying depending on the sensitivity of the test and the timing of testing with respect to missed menses, last intercourse, or last pregnancy.[15-17] For example, pregnancy tests are not able to detect a pregnancy resulting from recent intercourse, and pregnancy tests may remain positive several weeks after a pregnancy ends. The US SPR provides highly accurate criteria that a practitioner can review with a patient; in most cases, a detailed history provides the most accurate assessment of pregnancy risk. If a woman has no signs or symptoms of pregnancy and meets any one of the following criteria, a practitioner can be reasonably certain that the woman is not pregnant:

- if no more than 7 days after the start of normal menses
- has not had sexual intercourse since the start of last normal menses
- has been correctly and consistently using a reliable method of contraception
- is no more than 7 days after spontaneous or induced abortion
- is within 4 weeks postpartum
- is fully or nearly fully breastfeeding (exclusively breastfeeding or the vast majority [≥85%] of feeds are breastfeeds), amenorrheic, and less than 6 months postpartum

Routine pregnancy testing for every woman is not necessary. However, based on clinical judgment, a practitioner may consider the addition of a urine pregnancy test to rule out pregnancy, taking into account the limitations of pregnancy tests noted earlier. Emergency contraception may also be considered, if appropriate.

The next clinical consideration is whether the patient needs any examinations or tests before initiating the method. Although some examinations or tests may be needed, requiring unnecessary tests may be a barrier to starting contraception. For example, adolescents may not be comfortable with a pelvic examination. Waiting for test results may be another barrier associated with examinations and tests before initiating contraception. The US SPR[8] provides recommendations that address examinations and tests needed before a healthy woman starts a contraception method. The recommendations are categorized into 3 classes: (1) class A examinations and tests are essential and mandatory for a given method; (2) class B examinations and tests contribute substantially to safe and effective use, but implementation may be considered within the public health and/or service context; and (3) class C examinations and tests do not contribute substantially to safe and effective use of the method. These classifications focus on the relationship of the examinations and tests to safe initiation of a contraceptive method and are not intended to address the appropriateness of these examinations or tests in other circumstances (eg, for good preventive health care).

For the implant, no examinations or tests are needed. For other methods, there are very few class A examinations and tests. A bimanual examination and cervical inspection are essential before placement of an IUD, and a bimanual examination (not cervical inspection) is needed to fit a diaphragm or cervical cap; these are not needed for any other method. Based on CDC sexually transmitted diseases treatment guidelines,[14] screening for STIs should also be considered for women initiating IUDs and can be performed at the time of insertion. Although practitioners are encouraged to assess a patient's need for STI services during a family planning visit, screening for STIs is not necessary for safe initiation of other contraceptive methods.[18] A blood pressure examination is necessary before initiating CHCs, but the recommendation is accompanied by the following statement: in instances in which blood pressure cannot be measured by a health care professional, blood pressure measured in other settings can be reported by the woman to her practitioner.[8] For IUDs and hormonal methods, including the implant, the US SPR states that weight measurement and body mass index (BMI) calculation are not needed to determine medical eligibility; however, measuring weight and calculating BMI at baseline might be helpful for monitoring any changes and for counseling women who might be concerned about weight change perceived to be associated with the method. For women choosing a method of emergency contraception, emergency contraceptive pills might be less effective for women with obesity, but there are no safety concerns.

Routine follow-up after initiation of implants, or any contraceptive method, is generally not needed. However, practitioners are encouraged to advise patients to return at any time to discuss side effects or other problems, if the patient wants to change the method being used, and when it is time to remove or replace the contraceptive method (or for reinjection for DMPA users). Changes in bleeding patterns are one of the major reasons for discontinuation of contraception. If the patient returns and is experiencing irregular bleeding, the US SPR provides recommendations on anticipatory counseling for potential bleeding problems and proper management of women with bleeding irregularities while using contraception (eg, nonsteroidal anti-inflammatory drugs, hormonal treatment).

Clinical Scenario 3

A 17-year old, normal-weight female presents to your office. She reports unprotected intercourse 4 days ago and is worried about pregnancy.

Emergency contraception provides protection against pregnancy up to 120 hours after intercourse that occurs without any contraception or with a contraceptive failure (eg, missed pills, broken condom, or failed withdrawal). The 4 types of emergency contraception available in the United States are the Cu-IUD and 3 types of emergency contraceptive pills: ulipristal acetate (UPA), levonorgestrel (LNG) pills, and combined oral contraceptives (COCs), also known as the Yuzpe method.

Important considerations for emergency contraception include safety, effectiveness, access, and initiation of regular contraception. According to the US MEC, most women, including those with obesity, can safely use any of the emergency contraception methods. Emergency contraceptive pills will not cause an abortion or have teratogenic effects on the fetus if taken by a woman who is already pregnant. The Cu-IUD should not be used by a woman who is already pregnant (category 4) because of the risk for pelvic infection and septic spontaneous abortion.

The Cu-IUD is the most effective method of emergency contraception[8] and has the added benefit of providing long-term regular contraception; however, the method is only available from a trained provider. Although LNG pills are available over-the-counter for anyone of any age, UPA and COCs are available only by prescription, regardless of age. Ulipristal acetate has been shown to be more effective than LNG pills at and beyond 72 hours; LNG pills have been shown to be more effective than COCs and with fewer adverse effects.[8]

An important consideration when providing emergency contraception is also providing a regular method of contraception. According to the US SPR,[8] if a woman is starting regular contraception after taking UPA (an antiprogestin), the recommendation is to start or resume hormonal contraception no sooner than 5 days after taking UPA to avoid a potential interaction and decreased effectiveness of the emergency contraception. However, if the woman chooses a method that must be administered by a clinician (ie, IUD, implant, or DMPA) and therefore will require another visit, starting the method at the time of UPA initiation may be considered, weighing the risk of decreasing the effectiveness of UPA with the risk of not starting a regular contraceptive method. Regular contraception may be initiated at any time after starting LNG pills or COCs. The US SPR also recommends that an advance supply of emergency contraceptive pills be provided so that they are available when needed and can be taken as soon as possible after unprotected sex.

CONCLUSION

Rates of adolescent pregnancy in the United States are decreasing but remain high. Adolescents who are at risk for unintended pregnancy should have access to highly effective contraception. Health care professionals can use CDC contraception guidance to remove unnecessary medical barriers and increase adolescents' access to safe and effective contraception. Adolescents are medically eligible to use all methods of contraception based on age alone, although medical eligibility may differ for adolescents with certain medical conditions or other characteristics. Most females, including adolescents, can initiate contraception at any time (including the day of the visit) as long as the practitioner is reasonably certain that the woman is not pregnant. Few, if any, examinations or tests are needed before starting a contraceptive method. Because bleeding problems are a major reason for contraceptive discontinuation, the US SPR provides recommendations on anticipatory counseling for potential bleeding problems and proper management of bleeding. Routine follow-up after contraception initiation is generally not needed. However, practitioners are encouraged to advise patients to return at any time to discuss side effects or other problems, if the patient wants to change the method being used, and when it is time to remove or replace the contraceptive method (or for reinjection for DMPA users). Many options for emergency contraception are available to adolescents, including the Cu-IUD and different formulations of pills, after unprotected intercourse or as advance provision. Regular contraception should be started after emergency contraceptive in accordance with CDC guidance.

QUESTIONS

1. An adolescent has a medical condition and desires a method of contraception. You consult the U.S. Medical Eligibility Criteria for Contraceptive Use (US MEC) and determine that the contraceptive method is classified as a category 2 for this medical condition. This means that:
   A. There is no restriction for the use of the contraceptive method.
   B. The advantages of using the method generally outweigh the theoretical or proven risks.
   C. The theoretical or proven risks usually outweigh the advantages of using the method.
   D. There is an unacceptable health risk if the contraceptive method is used.
2. During an office visit, a 17-year-old requests initiation of the contraceptive implant today. She has no signs or symptoms of pregnancy, and her last menstrual period started 4 days ago. Which of the following statements is *true*?
   A. She needs a pregnancy test before having the implant placed.
   B. She needs to abstain from sex or use backup contraception for the next 7 days.

C. She can have the implant placed today.
D. She needs to have cervical cytology performed before undergoing implant insertion.

3. A 16-year-old has just started having sexual intercourse. After contraceptive counseling, she decides to initiate combined oral contraceptives (COCs). What examinations and tests are necessary before she can start taking COCs?
   A. Blood pressure measurement
   B. Clinical breast examination
   C. Bimanual examination
   D. Cervical cytology (Papanicolaou smear)
   E. Hemoglobin test
4. A 17-year-old had unprotected intercourse 4 days ago and is worried about pregnancy. What emergency contraception options can she use?
   A. Copper intrauterine device (Cu-IUD)
   B. Ulipristal acetate emergency contraceptive pills
   C. Levonorgestrel emergency contraceptive pills
   D. Combination estrogen/progestin pills
   E. All of the above
5. A 19-year-old has just requested emergency contraceptive pills (ECPs) and desires to start the combined vaginal ring as her regular method of contraception. How soon after taking ECPs can she start using the ring?
   A. If she chooses levonorgestrel ECPs, she can start the vaginal ring immediately. If she chooses ulipristal acetate ECPs, she should start the vaginal ring no sooner than 5 days after use of ECPs.
   B. At the time of her next menses
   C. After a negative pregnancy test
6. A sexually active 18-year-old reports that she has been using COCs consistently but wants to switch to a levonorgestrel IUD (LNG-IUD). She missed her last annual examination and has not been screened for sexually transmitted infections (STIs) in the past 12 months. She has no signs or symptoms of an STI. Can she start the LNG-IUD today?
   A. No, she needs to be screened for STIs and treated for any infection before she can receive an LNG-IUD.
   B. Yes. She can be screened for STIs today according to STI screening guidelines, and she also can receive an LNG-IUD. LNG-IUD placement should not be delayed.
   C. Yes, she can have the LNG-IUD, but she should be treated presumptively for chlamydial and gonococcal infection.

(See pages 196-197 for answers.)

References

1. Kost K, Maddow-Zimet I, Alex A. Pregnancies, Births and Abortions Among Adolescents and Young Women in the United States, 2013: National and State Trends by Age, Race and Ethnicity. New York: Guttmacher Institute; 2017
2. Sedgh G, Finer LB, Bankole A, Eilers MA, Singh S. Adolescent pregnancy, birth, and abortion rates across countries: levels and recent trends. *J Adolesc Health*. 2015;56(2):223-230
3. Dee DL, Pazol K, Cox S, Smith RA, et al. Trends in repeat births and use of postpartum contraception among teens—United States, 2004-2015. *MMWR Morb Mortal Wkly Rep*. 2017;66(16): 422-426
4. Lindberg L, Santelli J, Desai S. Understanding the decline in adolescent fertility in the United States, 2007-2012. *J Adolesc Health*. 2016;59(5):577-583
5. Trussell J. Contraceptive failure in the United States. *Contraception*. 2011;83(5):397-404
6. Martinez GM, Abma JC. Sexual activity, contraceptive use, and childbearing of teenagers aged 15-19 in the United States. *NCHS Data Brief*. 2015;209:1-8
7. Curtis KM, Tepper NK, Jatlaoui TC, et al. U.S. Medical Eligibility Criteria for Contraceptive Use, 2016. *MMWR Recomm Rep*. 2016;65(3):1-103
8. Curtis KM, Jatlaoui TC, Tepper NK, et al. U.S. Selected Practice Recommendations for Contraceptive Use, 2016. *MMWR Recomm Rep*. 2016;65(4):1-66
9. World Health Organization. *Medical Eligibility Criteria for Contraceptive Use*. Geneva: World Health Organization; 2015
10. World Health Organization. *Selected Practice Recommendations for Contraceptive Use*. 3rd ed. Geneva: World Health Organization; 2016
11. Mohllajee AP, Curtis KM, Flanagan RG, Rinehart W, Gaffield ML, Peterson HB. Keeping up with evidence a new system for WHO's evidence-based family planning guidance. *Am J Prev Med*. 2005;28(5):483-490
12. Hubacher D, Lara-Ricalde R, Taylor DJ, Guerra-Infante F, Guzman-Rodriguez R. Use of copper intrauterine devices and the risk of tubal infertility among nulligravid women. *N Engl J Med*. 2001;345(8):561-567
13. Jatlaoui TC, Simmons KB, Curtis KM. The safety of intrauterine contraception initiation among women with current asymptomatic cervical infections or at increased risk of sexually transmitted infections. *Contraception*. 2016;94(6):701-712
14. Workowski KA, Bolan GA; Centers for Disease Control and Prevention. Sexually transmitted diseases treatment guidelines, 2015. *MMWR Recomm Rep*. 2015;64(RR-03):1-137
15. Cervinski MA, Gronowski AM. Reproductive-endocrine point-of-care testing: current status and limitations. *Clin Chem Lab Med*. 2010;48(7):935-942
16. Cole LA. Human chorionic gonadotropin tests. *Expert Rev Mol Diagn*. 2009;9(7):721-747
17. Wilcox AJ, Baird DD, Dunson D, McChesney R, Weinberg CR. Natural limits of pregnancy testing in relation to the expected menstrual period. *JAMA*. 2001;286(14):1759-1761
18. Gavin L, Moskosky S, Carter M, et al; Centers for Disease Control and Prevention. Providing Quality Family Planning Services: Recommendations of CDC and the U.S. Office of Population Affairs. *MMWR Recomm Rep*. 2014;63(RR-04):1-54

Adolesc Med 030 (2019) 24–33

Incorporating the Adolescent in Individualized and Effective Contraceptive Counseling

Megan Jacobs, MD[a*]; Paritosh Kaul, MD[b]

[a]*Assistant Professor of Pediatrics, Adolescent Health and Medicine, Oregon Health and Science University, Doernbecher Children's Hospital, Portland, Oregon;* [b]*Professor of Pediatrics, Section of Adolescent Medicine, University of Colorado School of Medicine, Children's Hospital Colorado, Aurora, Colorado*

LEARNING OBJECTIVES

After reviewing this article, the reader should be able to perform the following in a contraceptive counseling visit with a patient:

1. Assess ways to maintain birth control confidentiality for each patient circumstance
2. Elicit patient priorities
3. Utilize motivational interviewing techniques
4. Propose individualized, evidence-based, and safe contraceptive options
5. Enumerate the role personal bias plays in contraceptive encounters

INTRODUCTION

Contraception and contraceptive counseling have evolved over time. Health care professionals ([HCPs], eg, physicians, physician assistants, social workers, health educators, nurses, and nurse practitioners) have also changed approaches to counseling in response to changes in society and technology. These methods have moved from primarily practitioner-dominated recommendations to a shared decision-making, patient-centered approach. The American Academy of Pediatrics recommends confidential sexual and reproductive health discussions

*Corresponding author
E-mail address: jacobsme@ohsu.edu

 ISSN 1934-4287

at each visit.[1] The HCPs sometimes struggle to make contraceptive counseling a priority because of perceived time constraints and lack of both standardized HCP knowledge and training.[2,3]

A thorough and individualized discussion about contraception might seem to be time-consuming, but a focused, patient-specific discussion can lead to efficient use of birth control (BC).[4] Additionally, female adolescents and young adults have been shown to improve their use of contraception and to be more satisfied with their BC if they choose their own method rather than one provided by their HCP.[5]

This article focuses on contraceptive counseling for female adolescents and young adults (hereafter referred to as *female adolescents*). There currently exists no single clear evidence-based method for contraceptive counseling; however, most current adolescent HCPs utilize evidence-based components, including individualized counseling, motivational interviewing (MI), and method-specific evidence. A thoughtful and individualized approach is necessary not only for patient autonomy but also for maintaining confidentiality, assessing female adolescent priorities, and obtaining informed consent. The article provides an evidence-based framework for enhancing the HCP's process of providing contraceptive counseling to female adolescents seeking BC. We will outline how to maintain confidentiality and assess patient priorities, and we propose an algorithmic discussion-tree based on the patient's personal history and desires for method choice. In addition, HCPs are encouraged to acknowledge potential personal biases in reproductive discussions and their effects on a young person's choice. Motivational interviewing will be introduced and encouraged as a pervasive concept to utilize in each contraceptive counseling visit. The proposed contraceptive counseling framework is outlined in Figure 1.

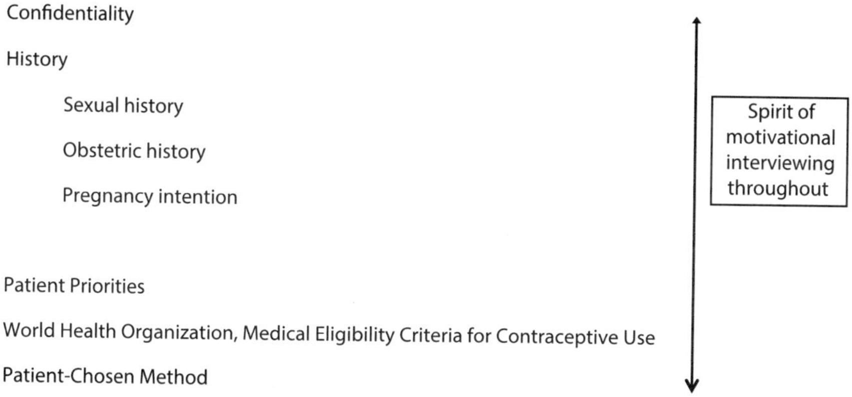

Fig 1. Contraceptive counseling framework.

By reframing the HCP mindset to empower the patient to become the expert on her own contraceptive choice, patient satisfaction and contraceptive method adherence will continue to improve.

Of note, although we acknowledge that contraceptive counseling can and should occur with all adolescent patients inclusive of all genders, anatomies, and sexual orientations, this article will focus primarily on anatomic females at risk for pregnancy and seeking contraception from an HCP.

THE SPIRIT OF MI

A successful conversation with an adolescent is one that involves trust, respect for the patient, and thoughtful listening. Motivational interviewing has been useful in producing adult and adolescent behavior change. Here we suggest applying MI strategies and principles outlined in the book by Miller and Rollnick[6] on MI to adolescent contraceptive counseling. This interviewing method has been effective in contraceptive uptake and use, and it has decreased rates of pregnancy at 1- to 2-year follow up.[7,8] The primary goal of contraceptive counseling is to assist female adolescents in making safe and well-informed personal choices about contraceptive options and not necessarily about writing a prescription. In contraceptive counseling, many tools of MI are extremely helpful in exploring patients' reproductive health desires and empowering them to make healthy and individualized contraceptive choices. The "spirit" of MI principles are summarized by the acronym PACE (Partnership, Acceptance, Compassion, Evocation).[6] The partnership is acknowledged by the interviewer by recognizing the adolescent as the expert on herself. Acceptance means supporting the patient's autonomy through verbal and non-verbal communication, such as listening to the full concern about a rumored adverse effect and then nodding, as opposed to interrupting the patient in an attempt to debunk a myth. Maintaining an active commitment to the patient's complete well-being demonstrates compassion. Finally, evoking the "how" and "why" of change, or decision-making in this case, is preferred over directing the patient with unsolicited advice. We recommend asking permission to share statistics or educational information with the adolescent before rattling off information without an invitation. Elements of MI with examples are reviewed in Table 1.

CONFIDENTIALITY

Confidentiality is vital for honest and comprehensive adolescent health care related to sensitive topics.[9] State laws and insurance issues affecting adolescent confidentiality are discussed in the article on policy foundations by Grubb and Upadhya in this issue of AM:STARs. Usually there is a point in a counseling visit when the patient and practitioner can speak privately to assess for other sexual health risk factors and possible coercion by a parent or sexual partner to influence an adolescent's decision regarding family planning.[10] If parents or sexual partners are perceived to be unsupportive of a patient's choice of BC, then some

Table 1
Motivational interviewing OARS strategies

Strategy	Examples
O (Open-ended questions)	HCP: *Tell me what you've heard about birth control.*
A (Affirmations)	Patient: *I have tried pills in the past but forgot to take them several times a month and had some irregular bleeding.*
	HCP: *It's difficult for most individuals to remember to take a pill every day.*
R (Reflections)	Patient: *I've taken Plan B 3 times in the last 2 months.*
	HCP: *It sounds like pregnancy is not something you are looking for right now.*
S (Summaries)	HCP: *It sounds like you are interested in a reliable birth control method to prevent pregnancy yet still have some questions about possible adverse effects.*

HCP, health care professional.
Derived from Miller WR, Rollnick S. *Motivational Interviewing: Preparing People for Change.* 3rd ed. New York: Guilford Press; 2013.

contraceptive methods, such as those that have amenorrhea-like effects or require a prescription, which could be discovered in the home, may not be optimal choices for an adolescent female. The HCP and the patient should discuss how the adolescent might handle these scenarios. With every contraceptive counseling visit, we recommend reviewing the adolescent's environmental and social safety regarding her potential BC method. For example, asking "Would anyone in your life be upset if they discovered you were using birth control?" is a good way to find out what the adolescent believes might be her parent's or partner's reaction to discovering the BC. An adolescent female in a relationship that has a threat of physical violence may be in danger if the partner discovers her use of contraception. Alternatively, the patient may be at risk of homelessness if parents discover contraceptive use by their daughter. Explicitly assessing for the level of confidentiality necessary is vital to the safety of the adolescent female and her adherence with her chosen contraceptive method.

HISTORY-TAKING

Obtaining an overview of the patient's health status is important for the HCP to counsel on safe and appropriate contraceptive methods. Medical, surgical, and family history should be reviewed. The U.S. Medical Eligibility Criteria for Contraceptive Use should be referenced for evidence-based contraindications and safety ratings of contraceptive methods for each patient medical condition and medication.[11]

Social, sexual, and obstetric histories should also be reviewed, as well as coercion regarding BC choice from a partner or parent, high-risk behaviors, and risk of contraception adverse effects. Table 2 gives examples of questions to elicit details of relevant histories. This conversation sets the tone for a discussion of the patient's reproductive life plan.

Table 2
Suggested history questions and assessment

Questions	Topics Assessed
Sexual history	
Are you attracted to men, women, or both?	Inquires about possible behaviors and level of STI/pregnancy risk
Are you currently dating or in a sexual relationship?	Assesses risk of pregnancy
Approximately how many sexual partners would you say you have had in the past 12 months?	Assesses high-risk behaviors, coercion, and risk of STIs
As far as you are aware, have you ever had an STI?	Assesses STI risk
Have you had a new partner since the last time you were tested for STIs?	Determines need for same-day STI screening
When was the last time you had sex without a condom or birth control?	In combination with last menstrual period, assesses likelihood of early luteal phase pregnancy
What percent of the time do you use condoms during sex?	Assesses STI and pregnancy risk; educational opportunity
Contraceptive history	
Which birth control methods have you used before?	Assesses contraceptive experience
Have you had problems with any birth control methods in the past?	Leads to patient priorities around future method choice
Gynecologic history	
How old were you when you had your first period?	Determines gynecologic age and likelihood of ovulatory cycles
What was the first day of your last menstrual period?	In combination with last unprotected sex, assesses likelihood of early luteal phase pregnancy
If >21 years old: *Have you had a Pap smear?*	Assesses need for cervical cancer screening at visit; may also address questions about human papilloma virus and vaccine
If Yes to previous Pap smear	Obtain result and date of last Pap smear
Obstetric history	
Have you ever been pregnant?	Helpful in both past and current family planning intentions
If Yes to previous pregnancy(s)	Assess outcomes of pregnancy(s) for both health of future pregnancies and intention to prevent

STI, sexually transmitted infection.

Reproductive Life Plan

Necessary for any conversation about contraception is understanding a young woman's perception of her ideal timing of pregnancy or whether she envisions herself being pregnant in the future. Start with an open, non-judgmental question, such as "Tell me about your thoughts about pregnancy in the future." If the patient is thinking about having children in the next 1 to 3 years, then discussing options that could fit her timeframe can help direct an initial conversation. If she does not want to become pregnant for at least 10 years or even at all, then discussing longer-lasting methods or higher-efficacy methods would be appropriate. Simply asking what the patient thinks might be a BC method to use until she is ready to become pregnant is another way to begin assessing the patient's overall knowledge of BC and her current mindset in her approach to pregnancy prevention.

PATIENT PRIORITIES

Needs Assessment

Based on history-taking of recent unprotected intercourse and date of last menstrual period, the HCP can estimate a patient's risk for a current early luteal phase pregnancy undetected by a urine pregnancy test ($<$10-14 days since conception) and can counsel on the potential need for emergency contraception the same day as the visit (if unprotected sex $\leq$5 days ago).

Patient-Driven Options

By asking the patient "What is the most important thing you'd like your birth control method to do for you?," the patient's autonomy is now established as the priority of the visit, and the HCP can avoid overwhelming the patient with a detailed list of all available BC methods. Many patients are seeking BC to prevent pregnancy but others may have different motives, so the HCP should be prepared to educate the patient on any beneficial effects of the available oral contraceptives. Providing examples can be very helpful, such as "Some of my patients feel like preventing pregnancy is the most important thing for them, but other patients use birth control to improve their acne, regulate their periods, or safely avoid having their periods, for example. Do any of those effects appeal to you as a reason to take birth control?"

Once the patient identifies her reason for wanting BC, then the HCP can begin discussing which option may work for her based on her health, priorities, and concerns (Table 3).

Table 3
Examples of possible patient priorities and concerns

Priorities for using birth control
Pregnancy prevention
Menstrual suppression
Acne treatment
Concerns about using birth control
Lowest hormones possible
Weight gain concerns
Mood concerns
Medication interaction concerns

Acknowledging the Patient's Perspective

Although many patients will already have an idea of which contraceptive method they would like to use, others will tell the HCP about personal experiences (or those of a friend) with contraception, good and bad. It is best to avoid invalidating a story, even if it sounds statistically or scientifically implausible. Instead, it is helpful to inquire whether the situation she is describing is of personal concern for her and whether she would like any additional data or information about possible adverse effects or fertility concerns. Figure 2 shows a contraceptive counseling algorithm.

Concluding the Visit

By the end of a contraceptive counseling visit, the patient may have chosen a contraceptive method. However, the HCP should also be willing to offer counseling for informational purposes only. Counseling should include explanations of ideal use, efficacy, safety, potential positive effects, and adverse effects. Visual aids and even videos can be helpful. Providing samples of an intrauterine device (IUD), implant, pill pack, ring, and patch models can be helpful for patients to feel and interact with throughout the decision-making and educational discussions. Table 4 lists some suggested online tools.

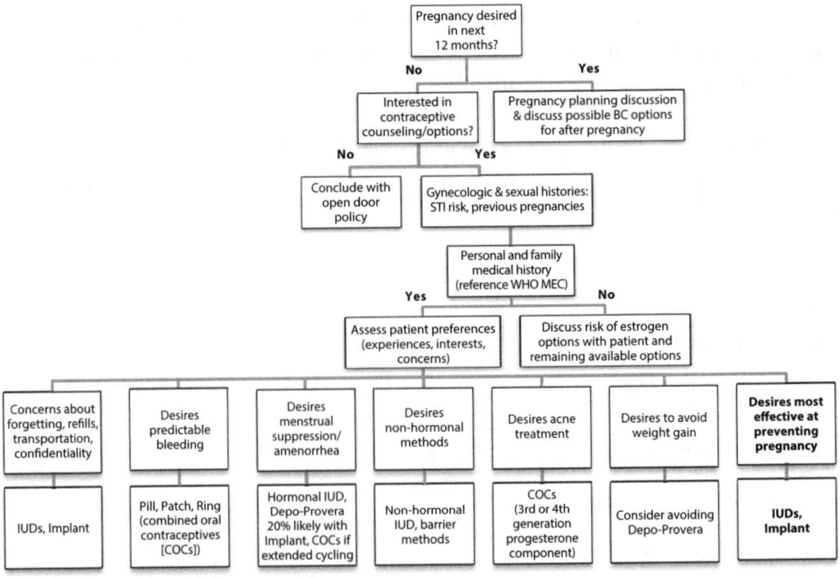

Fig 2. Contraceptive counseling algorithm.

Table 4
Decision-making and educational tools

Bedsider (https://bedsider.org)
Power to Decide (https://powertodecide.org/sexual-health/your-sexual-health/find-your-method; https://stayteen.org/videos)
To order on-hand office materials: https://shop.powertodecide.org/educational-materials/posters.html
Comprehensive Client-Center Contraceptive Counseling Resource Guide by Oregon Health Authority: https://www.oregon.gov/oha/PH/HealthyPeopleFamilies/ReproductiveSexualHealth/Documents/edmat/Client-CenterCounselingModelsandResources.pdf
Tia, a women's health advisor application (cycle, mood, and wellness tracker): https://asktia.com/app

Having an Open-Door Policy

The patient always has the right to change her mind at any time about her contraceptive method. As HCPs who care for adolescent females know, their patients can be impulsive and be subject to rapidly changing social and environmental factors leading to decision changes. We suggest acknowledging this by emphasizing that our goal as HCPs is to provide the patient with what she feels would be best for her in her life at the moment. If she goes home and feels that her choice may not have been the best for her, then she is always welcome to return and try other methods.

Practitioner Personal Bias

Unfortunately there is a history of governmental and clinician contraceptive coercion and sterilization in the United States.[12,13] Patients and their families can be hesitant to initiate contraception because of concerns about these past abuses of power over a women's reproductive health care. Although we do not assume that reproductive coercion is prevalent in current practices, we caution HCPs to reflect on even well-meaning personal biases. Public health concerns around teen pregnancy rates and associated negative health and social outcomes can motivate HCPs to attempt providing contraception to those who desire pregnancy.[14] Additionally, statistical evidence on highly efficacious methods such as hormonal implants and IUDs have influenced how some HCPs counsel their patients, perhaps persuading female adolescents to get an IUD when she may have preferred another method.[15] For example, a young woman with multiple sexual partners who has a history of pregnancy terminations and frequent emergency contraception use would like to start oral contraceptives because she is afraid of the pain and needles associated with longer-acting BC methods. It may be tempting to recommend long-acting reversible contraception as the best method for this patient because she is considered to be at high risk for unintended pregnancy. The patient's choice of a combined oral contraceptive pill may not provide her the most statistically effective method, but it might provide her with a higher level of control over her periods. Assessing the patient's priorities through the MI approach can validate the patient's decision or can expand her choice of contraceptive methods by offering relevant information. Matching the adolescent's priorities to the appropriate BC method will ultimately increase her satisfaction and adherence with her contraceptive method. The goal of the adolescent contraceptive counseling visit is to maintain the patient's autonomy. Thus, in the spirit of MI, effective counseling starts with the patient's concerns and ends with her possessing the knowledge to make an informed and personalized decision.

QUESTIONS

1. A 17-year-old female presents alone to your office for a contraceptive counseling visit. She admits to a lack of personal knowledge about her options. What might be a patient priority to explore at the visit today? Identify the best choice from the following options.
   A. How the patient thinks her family would react if she was on birth control
   B. Her plan, if any, to have children in the future
   C. The patient's concerns about her mental health
   D. All of the above
2. A 15-year-old female with whom you've been speaking about contraceptive options has used emergency contraception (EC) 3 times in the past 5 months and repeatedly reaffirms her choice of male condoms as her birth control method. Of the following options, choose the physician statement that is most consistent with a motivational interviewing approach.
   A. From your history of frequent EC use, it sounds like you are not interested in a long-acting form of birth control.
   B. Would it be alright if I asked what some of your likes and dislikes are about male condoms?
   C. It doesn't seem like male condoms work well for you and your partner. I think an arm implant or Depo-Provera shot might work better for you.
   D. If you're running out of condoms, I can write you a prescription for refills.
3. A 19-year-old female patient is trying to decide on a contraceptive method. Her history indicates that she had a blood clot during a previous pregnancy 2 years ago and has a body mass index of 35 kg/m^2. Her boyfriend does not want her to use birth control. Your patient does not want her boyfriend to find or feel her birth control, but she wants a very effective method. She also is attempting to lose weight and does not want her method to interfere with this goal. From the following options, which

would be the most ideal method for the patient when considering her health and wishes?

A. Arm implant
B. Copper intrauterine device (IUD)
C. Hormonal IUD
D. Depo-Provera injection
E. Vaginal ring

(See pages 198-199 for answers.)

References

1. Ott MA, Sucato GS; American Academy of Pediatrics Committee on Adolescence. Contraception for adolescents. *Pediatrics.* 2014;134(4):e1257-e1281
2. Bitzer J, Marin V, Lira J. Contraceptive counselling and care: a personalized interactive approach. *Eur J Contracept Reprod Health Care.* 2017; 22(6):418-423
3. Akers AY, Gold MA, Borrero S, Santucci A, Schwarz EB. Providers' perspectives on challenges to contraceptive counseling in primary care settings. *J Womens Health (Larchmt).* 2010;19(6): 1163-1170
4. Zapata LB, Tregear SJ, Curtis KM, et al. Impact of contraceptive counseling in clinical settings: a systematic review. *Am J Prev ed.* 2015;49(2 Suppl 1):S31-S45
5. Marcy SA, Brown JS, Danielson R. Contraceptive use by adolescent females in relation to knowledge, and to time and method of contraceptive counseling. *Res Nurs Health.* 1983;6(4):175-182
6. Miller WR, Rollnick S. *Motivational Interviewing: Preparing People for Change.* 3rd ed. New York: Guilford Press; 2013
7. Cowley CB, Farley T, Beamis K. "Well, maybe I'll try the pill for just a few months...": brief motivational and narrative-based interventions to encourage contraceptive use among adolescents at high risk for early childbearing. *Fam Syst Health.* 2002;20(2):183-204
8. Kirby D, Raine T, Thrush G, Yuen C, Sokoloff A, Potter SC. Impact of an intervention to improve contraceptive use through follow-up phone calls to female adolescent clinic patients. *Perspect Sex Reprod Health.* 2010; 42(4):251-257
9. Simmons M, Shalwitz J, Pollock S, Young A. *Adolescent Health Care 101: The Basics.* San Francisco, CA: Adolescent Health Working Group; 2003
10. Grace KT, Anderson JC. Reproductive coercion: a systematic review. *Trauma Violence Abuse.* 2018;19(4):371-390
11. Curtis KM, Tepper NK, Jatlaoui TC, et al. U.S. Medical Eligibility Criteria for Contraceptive Use, 2016. *MMWR Recomm Rep.* 2016;65(RR-3):1-104
12. Barot S. Governmental coercion in reproductive decision-making: see it both ways. *Guttmacher Policy Rev.* 2012;15(4):7-12
13. Benson Gold R. Guarding against coercion while ensuring access: a delicate balance. *Guttmacher Policy Rev.* 2014;17(3):8-14
14. Henderson JT, Raine T, Schalet A, Blum M, Harper CC. "I wouldn't be this firm if I didn't care": preventive clinical counseling for reproductive health. *Patient Educ Couns.* 2011;82:254-259
15. Gomez AM, Fuentes L, Allina A. Women or LARC first? Reproductive autonomy and the promotion of long-acting reversible contraceptive methods. *Perspect Sex Reprod Health.* 2014;46(3): 171-175

Adolesc Med 030 (2019) 34–44

New Approaches for Pregnancy Prevention: Getting Males Involved With Both Male- and Female-Dependent Methods of Contraception

Alexis Guzman, MD[a,b*]; David L. Bell, MD, MPH[a,b,c]

[a]*Department of Pediatrics, Columbia University College of Physicians and Surgeons, New York, New York;* [b]*New York Presbyterian Hospital, New York, New York;* [c]*Heilbrunn Department of Population and Family Health, Columbia University Mailman School of Public Health, New York, New York*

LEARNING OBJECTIVES

After reviewing this article, the reader should understand:

1. Male-dependent forms of contraception
2. How to get males more involved with female-dependent methods of contraception
3. The role that medical practitioners, parents, and others can play in helping males reduce unintended pregnancies

INTRODUCTION

Approximately 32.9% of pregnancies in the United States between 2011 and 2015 were unintended.[1] Despite numerous interventions primarily targeted toward women to reduce these unintended pregnancies, the rates continue to be high. Given the important health implications associated with unintended pregnancies for both the male and female involved, there has been a recent focus on getting adolescent and young adult males more involved with contraception, beyond male-dependent forms such as condom use. Getting adolescents to use contraception consistently, however, can be a complex and difficult process.

*Corresponding author
E-mail address: ag3888@cumc.columbia.edu

 ISSN 1934-4287

Lack of knowledge about contraception and its availability,[2] pressure from a partner to have sex,[3] the inability to communicate effectively,[4-8] and the influence of trust and commitment[9] are factors that can lead to inconsistent contraception use or nonuse.[10] The desire to have a child by either partner within a relationship may also strongly influence contraceptive use. This article will review how some of these factors play a role in how adolescent and young adult males can be involved in the prevention of unintended pregnancies. After reading this article, readers will understand male-dependent forms of contraception, how to get adolescent and young adult males more involved with female-dependent methods, and the role that medical practitioners, parents, and others can play in helping males reduce unintended pregnancies.

MALE-DEPENDENT METHODS OF CONTRACEPTION

Condoms

Condom use continues to be one of the most commonly used methods of contraception and is the only method that can prevent both pregnancy and the transmission of sexually transmitted infections (STIs). With real-life use, they are about 85% effective at preventing pregnancy (98% effective with perfect use). Condoms are made of rubber (latex), plastic (polyurethane, nitrile, or polyisoprene), or animal membranes, but only latex and synthetic condoms are recommended for the prevention of STIs.[11] Unfortunately, natural membrane condoms contain small pores that can allow the passage of viruses such as human immunodeficiency virus, hepatitis B, and herpes, making them less effective for STI protection.[12] In terms of their effectiveness for pregnancy prevention, typically latex condoms are the first to be recommended because some synthetic condoms may not prevent pregnancy as well or may break more often than condoms made of latex.[13] Condoms with the spermicide nonoxynol-9 are no longer recommended because they may increase the risk of human immunodeficiency virus transmission.[14] When counseling adolescent and young adult males about proper use of condoms, it is important to remind them to check the condom's expiration date, pinch the tip of the condom as they roll it on, hold the condom at the base of the penis when withdrawing after intercourse, and use only water- or silicone-based lubricants because oil-based lubricants can weaken latex condoms.

Numerous factors can affect patterns of condom use among adolescents, including relationship length and type, unequal power relations, use of hormonal contraceptives, the desire for pleasure, and limited sexual health education. Adolescent and young adult males in more committed relationships in which trust has been established are less likely to use condoms. Their use in these relationships can even be seen as a sign of infidelity by their partner.[15] In these relationships, condom use also declines when hormonal contraceptives are used because there is less worry about pregnancy prevention from the perspective of

related to pregnancy continuation or termination.[26] According to the Centers for Disease Control and Prevention, approximately 8.6% of women and 10.4% of men living in the United States have experienced pregnancy coercion.[27] While this type of coercion can be experienced by males and females, many sexual health programs have recognized the disparate power dynamics between men and women and have tried to address this problem by creating interventions that diminish the coercive behaviors of some men.[28] Appropriately discouraging coercive behaviors, however, is not at odds with encouraging supportive contraceptive behaviors and communication in the majority of relationships.

Male Involvement in Emergency Contraception

The last important topic to discuss with adolescent and young adult males regarding female-dependent methods is emergency contraception (EC) in the setting of unprotected sex, condom breakage or slippage, or contraceptive failure. In 2001, 48% of unintended pregnancies occurred during a month when contraceptives were used, likely a result of contraceptive failure or inappropriate use.[29] Therefore, it is important that males be informed about the EC methods available when unprotected sex or contraceptive failure occurs. These methods include the copper intrauterine device (ParaGard), ulipristal acetate (eg, ella), and levonorgestrel (eg, Plan B), from most effective to least effective.[30] Males should be told that all methods can be used up to 5 days after intercourse, but that Plan B is most effective when taken as early as possible after unprotected sex or contraceptive failure.

As with other contraceptive methods, there are barriers to EC access and use that must be overcome. Misconceptions about EC, such as it being an abortifacient or beliefs that it can affect an ongoing pregnancy, may be concerns that discourage use. The copper IUD and ella require seeing a doctor, and while ella can be requested on the Internet, an online medical consultation must be completed. Plan B, on the other hand, is available for purchase over the counter for all teens regardless of their age and has always been available for males and females to purchase. However, barriers to access do exist, as some teens may find it embarrassing to be seen purchasing it, may not have the money to do so, and pharmacies may impose unjustified barriers that are not in accordance with regulations.[31,32] Although the overall use of Plan B has not been shown to reduce pregnancy rates at the population level when given to females, advanced provision of it to females and males may help overcome barriers to use and increase access.[33] While it is a well-known practice to provide EC in advance to females, this is not the case for males. One study that evaluated advanced provision of EC to males found that 76% of males who were offered an EC package accepted it.[34] Until advanced provision of EC becomes a more common practice for males, they should be reminded that they are allowed to purchase Plan B at any pharmacy without a prescription and that if they are not able to do so they can always encourage their partner to obtain it through their medical practitioner.

ROLE OF MOTIVATIONAL INTERVIEWING TO INCREASE MALE INVOLVEMENT IN PREGNANCY PREVENTION

Changing health behaviors, including encouraging males to use condoms consistently and to be more involved with hormonal contraceptive use, is difficult to accomplish. Recently there has been a focus on using motivational interviewing (MI) to get patients to modify their lifestyles to more positive health behaviors (see article on incorporating the adolescent in individualized and effective contraceptive counseling by Kaul and Jacobs in this issue of AM:STARs). Through techniques such as the use of open-ended questions, affirmations, reflective listening, goal-setting, and summarizing, MI has been effective in improving numerous health behaviors and has been shown to reduce unintended pregnancies when used with adolescent females.[35,36] Its effectiveness in promoting behavioral change for the sexual and reproductive health of young males is currently being studied.[37] While awaiting results from this study and others, use of MI for reproductive health discussions with adolescent and young adult males in a clinical setting should be encouraged because its use may prove to play an important role in pregnancy prevention in the future.

CONCLUSION

Unintended pregnancy rates remain high and continue to take a toll on the health and socioeconomic development of our adolescents, which can affect not only their well-being but that of their families for years to come. Male involvement in contraception, including new approaches in which they take a more active role in use of hormonal methods, may provide an opportunity to reduce unintended pregnancies. To do this, adolescent and young adult males, like their female counterparts, should be taught about all forms of contraception, including the adverse effects, misconceptions, and barriers to use associated with them. Physicians, parents, and teachers should use their clinics, homes, schools, and other community-based settings to create an environment in which healthy and open discussions about sex and sexuality can take place. Teens and young adults must be encouraged to talk openly about contraception in these settings so that they may gain the communication skills needed to effectively negotiate safe sex with their partners and have the best chance of reaching their full potential as adults by reducing their risk of early parenthood.

QUESTIONS

1. An 18-year-old male presents to your adolescent medicine clinic for his annual physical examination. While providing his sexual history, he tells you that he has been sexually active with his girlfriend for the last 2 months. He uses condoms all of the time because his girlfriend is not using any birth control. He discloses that he is very anxious because about 2 days ago after having sex with his girlfriend, his condom slipped off while he was

pulling out of his partner's vagina. His girlfriend has not talked to her doctor about birth control or emergency contraception because she is scared her parents will find out she is having sex. He also discloses that his girlfriend always complains about heavy and painful periods. How do you best counsel this patient about the situation to reduce the risk of an unintended pregnancy?

A. His girlfriend should be seen by her medical practitioner to get a copper intrauterine device (ParaGard) because it is the most effective emergency contraceptive method and once placed will prevent pregnancy for 10 to 12 years.
B. The patient or his girlfriend should purchase levonorgestrel (Plan B) over-the-counter, and the girlfriend should take it as soon as possible.
C. His girlfriend should obtain ulipristal acetate (ella) through an online medical consultation and have it delivered to her overnight.

2. During a clinic visit for one of your 17-year-old male patients, his father privately discloses that his son has a girlfriend and he is concerned that his son is having or will have sex with her. He has not spoken to his son much about the matter because he had been hoping his son would delay having sex until he was older. In addition to wanting you to speak with his son about the matter, he wants you to tell him if his son is having sex so that he can try to provide him with more guidance. He also wonders what he can do to reduce his son's risk of a sexually transmitted infection (STI) and being involved in an unintended pregnancy. What advice do you provide this father with regard to his requests?
   A. Tell the father that you appreciate his concerns and that you will provide him with more information once you talk to the patient.
   B. Offer to discuss these issues with his son, remind the father about the confidentiality of your conversations with his son, and assure him that you both want to decrease his son's risk of an unintended pregnancy or an STI.
   C. Discuss some key points with father about condoms and contraception, answer any questions that he may have, and encourage him to speak with his son about these issues regardless of whether or not the patient is having sex.
   D. B and C

3. Which of the following statement(s) about condoms is *false*?
   A. They are the most commonly used method of contraception by adolescents.
   B. Natural membrane condoms contain small pores that allow transmission of viruses.
   C. They are the most effective male-dependent form of contraception.
   D. Condoms with the spermicide nonoxynol-9 may increase the risk of human immunodeficiency virus transmission.
   E. Only water- or silicone-based lubricants should be used with condoms.

4. A 16-year-old male presents to your clinic because he is interested in STI testing. He is currently sexually active with 1 female partner and states he uses condoms most of the time. When you ask him about whether his partner is using birth control, he tells you that he is not sure but that within a relationship he typically worries about the condoms and lets the girl worry about the birth control. How do you approach this situation?
   A. Congratulate him for using condoms most of the time and assess for any barriers to more consistent use.
   B. Discuss his short- and long-term life goals and how an unintended pregnancy could affect these goals.
   C. Tell him that his approach to pregnancy prevention is wrong and that if he continues to have this mindset he will likely get someone pregnant in the future.
   D. Ask him what he has heard about female-dependent methods of contraception and if he would be interested to learning more about them.
   E. Ask him if he has ever spoken to his partner about contraception, tell him that you invite him to consider speaking with her about it, and ask what would help him feel more comfortable to have that conversation.
   F. A, B, D, and E
   G. All of the above
5. A high school in your local community contacts you because they are interested in your help to improve the sexual and reproductive health of their students. They have a school-based health clinic that has recently seen an increase in students diagnosed with STIs and a few female patients who have gotten pregnant. They are interested in creating an educational curriculum for their students and clinical initiatives that could help reduce unintended pregnancies and STIs. What recommendations do you make to help improve the situation at their school?
   A. Discuss creating a sexual health curriculum that focuses on abstinence.
   B. Discuss creating a curriculum that focuses on teaching males about condom use and females about hormonal contraception.
   C. Discuss creating a curriculum that focuses on teaching all students about condoms and hormonal contraception.
   D. Discuss providing free condoms to all students at the school and clinical care that improves access to hormonal contraception, including long-acting reversible contraception.
   E. C and D

(See pages 199-200 for answers.)

References

1. Key statistics from the National Survey of Family Growth. Centers for Disease Control and Prevention. https://www.cdc.gov/nchs/nsfg/key_statistics/i.htm#intended
2. Ingham R. *Young People's Sex Advice Services: Delays, Triggers and Contraceptive Use*. Southampton: Centre for Sexual Health Research: University of Southampton; 2000
3. Dickson N, Paul C, Herbison P, Silva P. First sexual intercourse: age, coercion, and later regrets reported by a birth cohort. *BMJ*. 1998;316(7124):29-33
4. Coleman L, Ingham R. Attenders at young people's clinics in Southampton: variations in contraceptive use. *Br J Fam Plann*. 1998;24(3):101-104
5. Donald M, Lucke J, Dunne M, O'Toole B, Raphael B. Determinants of condom use by Australian secondary school students. *J Adolesc Health*. 1994;15(6):503-510
6. Hillier L, Harrison L, Warr D. "When you carry condoms all the boys think you want it": negotiating competing discourses about safe sex. *J Adolesc*. 1998;21(1):15-29
7. Shoop DM, Davidson PM. AIDS and adolescents: the relation of parent and partner communication to adolescent condom use. *J Adolesc*. 1994;17(2):137-148
8. Lear D. Sexual communication in the age of AIDS: the construction of risk and trust among young adults. *Soc Sci Med*. 1995;41(9):1311-1323
9. Aggleton C, Oliver C, Rivers K. *Reducing the Rate of Teenage Conceptions: the Implications of Research into Young People, Sex, Sexuality and Relationships*. London: Health Education Authority; 1998
10. Stone N, Ingham R. Factors affecting British teenagers' contraceptive use at first intercourse: the importance of partner communication. *Perspect Sex Reprod Health*. 2002;34(4):191-197
11. Lytle CD, Routson LB, Seaborn GB, Dixon LG, Bushar HF, Cyr WH. An in vitro evaluation of condoms as barriers to a small virus. *Sex Transm Dis*. 1997;24(3):161-164
12. Carey RF, Lytle CD, Cyr WH. Implications of laboratory tests of condom integrity. *Sex Transm Dis*. 1999;26(4):216-220
13. Gallo MF, Grimes DA, Lopez LM, Schulz KF. Non-latex versus latex male condoms for contraception. *Cochrane Database Syst Rev*. 2006;(1):CD003550
14. Centers for Disease Control and Prevention. Nonoxynol-9 Spermicide Contraception Use—United States, 1999. *MMWR Morb Mortal Wkly Rep*. 2002;51(18):389-392
15. Raine TR, Gard JC, Boyer CB, et al. Contraceptive decision-making in sexual relationships: young men's experiences, attitudes and values. *Cult Health Sex*. 2010;12(4):373-386
16. Manlove J, Ikramullah E, Terry-Humen E. Condom use and consistency among male adolescents in the United States. *J Adolesc Health*. 2008;43(4):325-333
17. Pleck J, Sonenstein F, Ku L. Masculinity ideology: its impact on adolescent males' heterosexual relationships. *J Soc Issues*. 1993;49(3):11-29
18. Blake SM, Ledsky R, Goodenow C, Sawyer R, Lohrmann D, Windsor R. Condom availability programs in Massachusetts high schools: relationships with condom use and sexual behavior. *Am J Public Health*. 2003;93(6):955-962
19. Horner JR, Salazar LF, Romer D, et al. Withdrawal (coitus interruptus) as a sexual risk reduction strategy: perspectives from African-American adolescents. *Arch Sex Behav*. 2009;38(5):779-787
20. Rayala BZ, Viera AJ. Common questions about vasectomy. *Am Fam Physician*. 2013;88(11): 757-761
21. Guzman BL, Schlehofer-Sutton MM, Villanueva CM, Stritto MED, Casad BJ, Feria A. Let's talk about sex: how comfortable discussions about sex impact teen sexual behavior. *J Health Commun*. 2003;8(6):583-598
22. Coleman LM, Ingham R. Exploring young people's difficulties in talking about contraception: how can we encourage more discussion between partners? *Health Educ Res*. 1999;14(6):741-750
23. Catallozzi M, Bell DL, Short MB, Marcell AV, Ebel SC, Rosenthal SL. Does perception of relationship type impact sexual health risk? *Sex Transm Dis*. 2013;40(6):473-475

24. Merkh RD, Whittaker PG, Baker K, Hock-Long L, Armstrong K. Young unmarried men's understanding of female hormonal contraception. *Contraception.* 2009;79(3):228-235
25. Carter MW, Bergdall AR, Henry-Moss D, Hatfield-Timajchy K, Hock-Long L. A qualitative study of contraceptive understanding among young adults. *Contraception.* 2012;86(5):543-550
26. Miller E, Silverman JG. Reproductive coercion and partner violence: implications for clinical assessment of unintended pregnancy. *Exp Rev Obstet Gynecol.* 2010;5(5):511-515
27. Black M, Basile K, Breiding M, et al. *The National Intimate Partner and Sexual Violence Survey: 2010 Summary Report.* Atlanta, GA: National Center for Injury Prevention and Control, Centers for Disease Control and Prevention; 2011
28. Sternberg P, Hubley J. Evaluating men's involvement as a strategy in sexual and reproductive health promotion. *Health Promot Int.* 2004;19(3):389-396
29. Finer LB, Henshaw SK. Disparities in rates of unintended pregnancy in the United States, 1994 and 2001. *Perspect Sex Reprod Health.* 2006;38(2):90-96
30. Batur P, Kransdorf LN, Casey PM. Emergency Contraception. *Mayo Clinic Proceedings.* 2016; 91(6):802-807
31. Marcell AV, Waks AB, Rutkow L, McKenna R, Rompalo A, Hogan MT. What do we know about males and emergency contraception? A synthesis of the literature. *Perspect Sex Reprod Health.* 2012;44(3):184-193
32. Wilkinson TA, Clark P, Rafie S, Carroll AE, Miller E. Access to emergency contraception after removal of age restrictions. *Pediatrics.* 2017;140(1):e20164262
33. Polis CB, Schaffer K, Blanchard K, Glasier A, Harper CC, Grimes DA. Advance provision of emergency contraception for pregnancy prevention (full review). *Cochrane Database Syst Rev.* 2007;(2):CD005497
34. Garbers S, Bell DL, Ogaye K, Marcell AV, Westhoff CL, Rosenthal SL. Advance provision of emergency contraception to young men: an exploratory study in a clinic setting. *Contraception.* 2018;98(2):106-109
35. Lundahl B, Moleni T, Burke BL, et al. Motivational interviewing in medical care settings: a systematic review and meta-analysis of randomized controlled trials. *Patient Educ Couns.* 2013;93(2): 157-168
36. Barnet B, Liu J, DeVoe M, Duggan AK, Gold MA, Pecukonis E. Motivational intervention to reduce rapid subsequent births to adolescent mothers: a community-based randomized trial. *Ann Fam Med.* 2009;7(5):436-445
37. Bell DL, Garbers S, Catallozzi M, et al. Computer-assisted motivational interviewing intervention to facilitate teen pregnancy prevention and fitness behavior changes: a randomized trial for young men. *J Adolesc Health.* 2018;62(3S):S72-S80

Adolesc Med 030 (2019) 45–59

Condoms On and Off: A Review of Prophylactic Barrier Use and Youth Sexual Well-Being

J. Dennis Fortenberry, MD, MS

Department of Pediatrics, Division of Adolescent Medicine, Indiana University School of Medicine, Indianapolis, Indiana

Barriers remain an essential, developmentally relevant element to prevention of sexually transmitted infections for most youth. In particular, barriers can be flexibly implemented to a variety of sexual behaviors that reflect diverse partners' preferences as well as sexual and gender identities. However, barriers continue to represent a broad challenge to the beliefs of many young people about sexual trust and intimacy. The objective of this review is to provide an evidence-based understanding of the role of barriers in the sexual well-being of contemporary youth, with emphasis on sexual relationships, sexual function, and pleasure.

LEARNING OBJECTIVES

After reviewing the article, the reader should be able to:

1. List at least 3 modes of sex for which barriers may be useful
2. Describe the role of trust in decision-making about barrier use
3. Summarize arguments for and against the role of barriers in youth's sexual pleasure

INTRODUCTION

This review of prophylactic barrier use and sexual well-being among adolescents and young adults emphasizes the importance of barriers in the sexual behaviors of youth. Particular attention is given to relational and symbolic meanings of barriers in youth sexuality, sex, fertility, and sexually transmitted infections (STIs).

E-mail address: jfortenb@iu.edu

 ISSN 1934-4287

This symbolism is key to public health and clinical issues relevant to youths' sexual well-being, most centrally the relational trust and intimacy that are prioritized in American sexual mythology. The review is organized by an "on/off" metaphor, referring simultaneously to ambivalence of decisions to use barriers (especially barriers designed to cover an erect penis) in specific relational contexts, the intermittent nature of barrier use for many youth, the mechanics of barrier use in multiple types of sexual interaction, and the odd but defining contemporary term: condomless sex.

The review is focused on barrier use with specific modes of sex. Emphasis is given to public health and clinically relevant, peer-reviewed, English-language, and United States (US)-focused research published during the past 5 years. This is a narrative rather than systematic review; however, the volume of published research precludes comprehensive inclusion, and many papers are cited that fail 1 or more of the selection criteria to more thoroughly address specific issues. The overall objective of the review is to support a broad evidence-based understanding of the role of barriers in the sexual well-being of contemporary youth, with particular emphasis on sexual relationships, sexual function, and pleasure.

NOMENCLATURE USED IN THIS REVIEW

The term *youth* is used here to refer to a socially relevant period roughly corresponding to the second and third decades of life, extending a developmental period between childhood and adulthood from puberty to age 24.[1] When needed for developmental relevance, *adolescents* refer to those aged 17 and younger and *young adults* to those aged 18 and older. Literature that gives detailed focus on barrier use by younger adolescents (14 years and younger) is particularly limited and will be identified as associated with early adolescence.

Traditional categories of American race/ethnicity will not be used as a lens for understanding youth barrier use, although small-to-modest, consistent group differences have been identified in population-focused surveys.[2] The rationale for rejecting these traditional categories here is that emphasis on race/ethnicity group differences blurs the focus on sexuality and relationships and underemphasizes large within-group diversity in sexual behaviors and barrier use that is of far greater clinical and public health importance than between-group differences. For example, no single racial/ethnic group uniformly rejects or accepts barriers for young people.[3] Race/ethnicity-based barrier use interventions likely benefit from cultural, social, gender, religious, and linguistic adaptations that contribute to intergroup race/ethnicity differences, but these tailored programs do not depend on understanding intergroup differences in barrier use for effective implementation.

In terms of traditional gender and sexual identity categories, there is no widely accepted professional language to differentiate barrier use currently named for

Table 1
Barrier types, coverage, and mode of sex

Usual barrier name	Anatomic site coverage	Mode of sex
Condom[a] (latex, polyurethane, natural)	Penis	Penis–vulva/vagina Penis–anus/rectum Penis–mouth/lips/tongue/pharynx Sex toy–vulva/vagina Sex toy–anus/rectum Sex toy–lips/mouth/tongue/pharynx
Female condom[b] (latex, nitrile, polyurethane)	Vulva/vagina/cervix Anus/rectum	Vulva/vagina–penis Anus/rectum–penis
Dental dam (latex, various plastics)	Vulva Anus	Vulva–mouth/lips/tongue Anus–mouth/lips/tongue
Gloves (latex, nitrile)	Finger(s)/hand	Finger/hand–vulva/vagina Finger/hand–anus/rectum

[a] *Condom* unmodified by a gender term refers to a penis-covering barrier.
[b] *Female condom* refers to a condom designed for intravaginal use even if used for anus/rectum coverage by males.

binary sex/gender classifications (eg, terms such as *female* and *male* condoms) from barrier use by people with diverse sexual and gender identities and genital configurations. For example, birth-assigned females may cover sex toys with a *male* barrier during sex with another birth-assigned female, and birth-assigned males may use a *female* barrier for anal/rectal sex. Men with a vulva/vagina/cervix and women with a penis/testicles both use gender-labeled barriers according to anatomy and mode of sex, not sex assigned at birth.

To emphasize barriers as genderless and sexless, explicit nomenclature has been used to differentiate penis-covering barriers (usually identified as *male condoms* or simply *condoms*) from those for vulva/vagina/cervix covering (identified and marketed as *female* condoms and never simply *condoms*), and both are differentiated from those for vulva or anus/rectum covering (Table 1). Use of sexual identity and behavior description terms such as *gay/straight/lesbian/bisexual*, *women-who-have-sex-with-women-and-men*, and *men-who-have-sex-with-men* have been avoided to ground barrier use as components of specific modes of sex rather than imprecise attributes of various sexual or gender identity categories.

BARRIER USE FOR MODE-SPECIFIC SEX

Four modes of sex relevant to barriers are addressed: penis and vulva/vagina; penis and anus/rectum; penis and lips/mouth/tongue/pharynx; and lips/mouth/tongue and vulva/vagina or anus. When appropriate, the anatomic site(s) covered by a specific type of barrier is named first, then the partner's corresponding anatomic site(s) of the particular mode of sex (Table 1). These relatively exact anatomic terms are used to avoid prioritizing specific forms of sex such as penis–vulva/vagina sex, which is often understood simply as *sex* or even *regular* or *normal* sex. Modes of sex such as finger/hand–genital/anus, lips/mouth/tongue–anus, and sex toy–genital/anus have a limited empirical literature for review but are mentioned for completeness. A limitation of this mode-specific approach to barrier use categorization is the likelihood of multiple modes of sexual activities within a single sexual interaction,[4,5] but this is unavoidable given the limits of existing research literature that prioritizes specific modes of sex such as penis–vulva/vagina and penis–anus/rectum.

Penis-Covering Barriers

Rates of use of penis-covering barriers during penis–vulva/vagina sex are high for first partnered experiences: up to 80% or more,[6,7] depending on the data source. These levels may not be maintained during subsequent experiences, even with different (new) partners. Rates of up to 80% at most recent experience are reported, as well as rates of 50% or less.[8-11] There are some important developmental points: barrier use at first experience is lower among younger (14 years or younger) than older (17-19 years) adolescents but are higher at most recent experience for younger (9th grade) than older (12th grade) adolescents.[2,6,12] Rates of dual-method use (defined here as joint barrier/contraceptive use rather than other dual-method use options such as joint barrier/preexposure prophylaxis use[13]) are highest for the combination of barrier plus oral contraceptives and lowest for those using long-acting reversible methods.[2,14,15] Barrier use is also higher (~60%) in physical contexts such as parked cars, which may be especially relevant to youth who do not have access to private personal space.[16] Rates of barrier use are affected by embarrassment, as electroencephalographic P300 event-related potentials demonstrate early attentional disengagement among those with embarrassment about barrier purchase, even among those endorsing a high behavioral intention to use barriers.[17] Use is not simply a matter of individual preference; youth who might consider penis-covering barrier use face multiple obstacles, such as abstinence-only school education programs that restrict knowledge, diminish social acceptability, and limit physical access to barriers within school clinics.[18,19] Free or low-cost distribution programs are cost-effective, although evidence of communitywide effectiveness for prevention of human immunodeficiency virus (HIV) infection is still lacking.[20,21] Under multiple assumptions of uptake and effectiveness, worldwide, penis-covering barriers are cost-effective.[22,23]

Four issues should be considered in understanding youth's penis-covering barrier use: (1) semen exposure; (2) fit and feel of penis-covering barriers; (3) barrier use problems and errors; and (4) relationships, sexual pleasure, and sexual function issues associated with penis-covering barriers.

Semen Exposure

The apparently self-evident importance of semen exposure associated with penis-covering barriers has several interesting twists. First, the best interpretation of barrier use self-reports in recent sexual experiences is open to question. For example, Y chromosome assay (as a marker of intravaginal semen presumably associated with penis–vulva/vaginal sex with ejaculation without use of a penis-covering barrier) was positive among 63 of 186 15- to 21-year-olds who reported 100% barrier use during penis–vulva/vagina sex.[24] Second, semen modifies a variety of immune responses in rectal and vaginal tissues. For example, penis–anus/rectum sex is associated with rectal immune cellular phenotypes and proinflammatory cytokines associated with mucosal injury and repair.[25] Third, penis-covering barriers are linked to multiple stages of human papillomavirus (HPV) oncogenesis, including high-risk HPV infection, infection persistence, and development/regression of cervical intraepithelial neoplasia, and may be relevant to more than simple infection prevention.[26-31] Fourth, semen is viewed by some as a marker of relationship and sexual intimacy and exclusivity (*fluid bonded*), or the erotic elements of semen or "cum" play.[32,33] Even when penis-covering barriers are in place during most of a sexual event, ejaculation may occur with the barrier removed. In those circumstances, ejaculation may occur on the partner's body or elsewhere, such as a towel or bedsheet.[34]

Fit and Feel

The appropriate matching of penis-covering barriers and penis dimensions (*fit*) improves user sexual satisfaction (*feel*) and reduces breakage and slippage. Break/slip rates of 10% to 30% are reported among youth but may be higher among those less experienced in barrier use and among people living with HIV.[35,36] Penis size is associated with breakage of penis-covering barriers, especially with penis–anus/rectum sex.[36-41] Of potential relevance to younger adolescents are the changes in flaccid penile length that continue during puberty through genital stage 5, and circumference change may continue even longer.[42,43] Thus, the fit of penis-covering barriers—like that of shoe size and other clothing—may change over development time and require periodic reassessment.

Barrier Use Problems and Errors

The idea that effective use of penis-covering barriers requires knowledge and technical skill has been around for years.[36,44] The technical issues accompanying effective use of penis-covering barriers includes application after starting sex and removal before ejaculation, difficulty with packaging or condom orientation on the penis, and issues with lubrication and dryness.[44-46] Data addressing these problems and errors were thoroughly reviewed in 2012 by Sanders et al.[47] The frequency of barrier use problems and errors is associated with STI risk.[48-50] Brief interventions to improve technical capacity in barrier use can be effective,[51] but these kinds of practical skills-building trainings are not typically used in school-based programs designed for adolescents.[52]

Relationships, Sexual Pleasure, and Sexual Function

Almost from the beginning of the US HIV epidemic in the early 1980s, efforts to promote penis-covering barrier use by youth have been confronted by the symbolic contradiction of barriers to the trust, intimacy, and commitment elements intrinsic to sexual and romantic ideologies focused on monogamy.[53-55] Barrier use after the early weeks or months of a sexual relationship continues to be seen as unnecessary and contradictory in the context of a committed relationship.[56-58] In particular, trust—as an alternative to barriers in the context of a trustworthy, monogamous partner—is viewed by partners as an effective infection prevention practice that is often resistant to counterevidence of relationship infidelity.[59] More successful interventions to improve barrier use now attempt to account for competing priorities within those relationships, especially in terms of trust, intimacy, and relationship maintenance motivations.[57,60]

Many youth have a broad perception of penis-covering barriers as antithetical to pleasure.[61-63] Even early adolescents without partnered sexual experiences express negative attitudes about penis-covering barriers, related to interference with pleasure.[64] Young adults perceive penis–vulva/vagina sex as more pleasurable without penis-covering barriers, although these differences are largely a function of relationship status.[61] This is not a uniform perception, however. For example, about 25% of youth report enhanced pleasure associated with penis-covering barrier use for penis–anus/rectum sex,[65] and some studies found no difference in reported pleasure associated with penis-covering barrier use for penis–vulva/vagina sex.[66]

As with much of developmental sexuality, development of the physiologic and neurocognitive elements of sexual arousal, penis sensation and erectile response, vaginal lubrication, and orgasm are all poorly understood among peri- and post-pubertal adolescents, especially as these sexual functions intersect with use of penis-covering barriers. Some research is emerging, however. Although both implicit and explicit attitudes of youth toward penis-covering barriers are relevant to barrier use under conditions of sexual arousal, implicit attitudes are relatively more influential during sexual arousal and penile erection.[67,68] This is thought to be the result of elements of executive functioning, such as inhibition and working memory, which are highly utilized during arousal and may be especially limited cognitive resources during early and middle adolescence.[69-71] An implication of this type of work would be more developmentally relevant barrier use interventions focused on implicit attitudes and youth's developing executive functions.

Other clinically relevant issues of penis-covering barriers include erectile dysfunction, pain, and discomfort. Persistent sexual problems such as erectile dysfunction are not rare among young people,[72] and for up to 50% these problems are persistent.[73] Erectile dysfunction is an important correlate of non-use of penis-covering barriers and may be associated with non-prescribed use of medications such as sildenafil and other phosphodiesterase type 5 inhibitors.[74-76] Vulvar/vaginal/pelvic pain associated with penis–vulva/vagina sex is common,[77,78] perhaps more so with penis-covering barriers.[49] Many youth respond to barrier-related sexual dysfunctions simply by abandoning their use, but there seem to be no data addressing the efficacy of other interventions to sustain youth's penis-covering barrier use in the context of experiences of sexual dysfunction.

Penis-Covering Barriers in Penis–Lips/Mouth/Tongue/Pharynx Sex

As with other modes of sex, penis–lips/mouth/tongue/pharynx sexual experiences become more prevalent with age. Among 6th- to 8th-graders, about 5% report lifetime experience.[79] About 39% of American adolescents aged 15 to 19 years and more than 70% of young adults aged 20 to 24 years (all reporting on sexual events with different sex partners) report lifetime experience giving or receiving penis–lips/mouth/tongue sex. Penis-covering barrier use at last penis–lips/mouth/tongue/pharynx sex is about 10% and 7% for 15- to 19-year-olds and 20- to 24-year-olds, respectively.[80-82] Improved understanding of the public health importance of extragenital STI is leading to a renewed need to understand barrier use for lips/mouth/tongue/pharynx modes of sex. For example, increased barrier use could reduce the prevalence of some oropharyngeal STIs.[83] Among other needs for consideration of a sexual health perspective in approaching youth barrier use, it would be useful to frame new dialogues outside of the "moral panic" expressions that accompanied previous explorations of penis–lips/mouth/tongue/pharynx sex among adolescents,[84] promoting a less heteronormative perspective and recognizing youths' diverse positive and negative experiences with this mode of sex.[85-87]

Penis- and Anus/Rectum-Covering Barriers in Penis–Anus/Rectum Sex

Lifetime rates of penis–anus/rectum sex increase with age: 11% among 15- to 19-year-olds and 32% to 34% among 20- to 24-year-olds.[80] Rates of penis-covering barrier use at first and most recent penis–anus/rectum sex vary from just less than 50% to more than 85%, depending on sexual position and HIV serostatus. The rates of penis–anus/rectum sex without a penis-covering barrier have always been relatively low for different sex dyads but seem to have decreased during the past decade.[88,89] Reasons for the trend away from barrier use for penis–anus/rectum sex include relational intimacy and monogamy, generational prevention fatigue, widespread use of antiretroviral therapy, and preexposure prophylaxis.[90-92] Recent innovations in individual communication technology and mHealth (mobile health) interventions have not yet fulfilled expectations for more widespread use of penis-covering barrier use among youth.[93] Although lack of penis-covering barrier use at first penis–anus/rectum sex is associated with subsequent HIV/STI risk behavior, sexual and emotional satisfaction are not.[94] Relatively little is known about the developmental trajectories of penis-covering barrier use and seroadaptive behaviors such as serosorting, seropositioning, and viral load sorting, although it is clear that the intersection of partners' HIV infection statuses, or of viral load, are important contexts of penis-covering barrier use for penis–anus/rectum modes of sex.[95-98] Failure of penis-covering barriers to prevent HIV transmission may be more significant than acknowledged. One study identified 51% of new HIV transmissions were associated with penis–anus/rectum sex using a penis-covering barrier.[99]

Anus/rectum-covering barriers for anus/rectum–penis modes of sex involve anal insertion of devices approved by the US Food and Drug Administration only as vulva/vagina/cervix barriers. Uncertainty remains about appropriate use for anus/rectum–penis sex.[100,101] Slippage and pain are both reported with this use,[102] but some endorse their use. No data address the efficacy, safety, and functionality of newer barrier designs, especially among younger users.

Vagina/Vulva-Covering Barriers in Vulva/Vagina–Penis Sex

These barriers (identified as *female* condoms) are designed to cover the cervix, vagina, and portions of the vulva. Several similar designs are available internationally, but only 1 is marketed in the United States.[103] These barriers consist of an inner and outer ring at each end, is 170 mm in length, and is made of synthetic nitrile latex with silicone lubricant. Rates of use at most recent sex are less than 10%,[104] and few recent studies have specifically addressed issues such as dual use or use by adolescents. However, vaginal/vulva-covering barriers are cost-effective for HIV prevention in higher risk populations,[105] have high rates of reimbursement,[106] and are amenable to brief interventions for both initial and sustained use.[107] Device failure rates (breakage, invagination, misdirection, and slippage) are reported around 5% and decrease with user experience.[103,108]

Vulva/Vagina-Covering Barriers in Vulva–Lips/Mouth/Tongue Sex

More explicit understanding of barriers for vulva–lips/mouth/tongue sex is increasingly important as the epidemiology of pharyngeal STI is better understood. These barriers are unappealingly and misleadingly identified as *dental dams*, and use seems to be routinely but unenthusiastically endorsed in STI/HIV prevention education.[109] Levels of use (especially consistent use) are low, and evidence of their effectiveness or even the best materials is lacking.[110-112] Misperceptions of these barriers, notably identification as female condoms, may additionally interfere with uptake.[113] Few data address understanding and use of these barriers by youth.

DISCUSSION

Prophylactic barriers are easy to put on and take off, are well known to many successive birth cohorts of US youth, are adaptable to a variety of modes of partnered sexual interaction, are relatively low cost, and are effective (although imperfect) for pregnancy and STI prevention. However, the literal essence of barriers to form an impermeable wall during sex is the basis for a widespread symbolic interpretation of barriers as antithetical to the trust and intimacy—and to sexual function and pleasure—that justify a romantic basis for non-reproductive sex, especially for youth.[55,56]

The most important "barrier" to use, however, has less to do with the physical forms of prophylactic barriers and more to do with youth sexuality as fiercely contested threads woven into the social, religious, and political fabric of American life. This remains especially relevant as key elements of young people's sexual learning is framed in abstinence-only until-marriage dialogues that censor fact-based content, discussion, and education about barriers. Public health science and policy, as well as clinical practice, are ethically bound to offer perspectives based in principles of evidence-based review. Pediatricians, as developmental health experts and youth advocates, can endorse comprehensive, sex-positive sexuality education (which includes barriers-related discussion and skills-building for negotiation and use) for all youth, as well as public health policies and clinical practices that promote youths' sexual health and sexual well-being.

QUESTIONS

1. What is the approximate rate of penis-covering barrier use at first partnered sex?
   A. 12%
   B. 40%
   C. 50%
   D. 80%
2. Penis size is unrelated to slippage/breakage of penis-covering barriers.
   A. False
   B. True
3. Sexual dysfunctions associated with youth penis-covering barrier use
   A. is rare because youth's cognitive executive function is fully developed.
   B. is rare because penile erectile function is maximal just after puberty.
   C. is associated with vulvar and vaginal pain in some users.
   D. always can be alleviated with use of appropriate lubricants.

(See page 200 for answers.)

References

1. Scales PC, Benson PL, Oesterle S, Hill KG, Hawkins JD, Pashak TJ. The dimensions of successful young adult development: a conceptual and measurement framework. *Appl Dev Sci.* 2016;20: 150-174
2. Steiner RJ, Liddon N, Swartzendruber AL, Rasberry CN, Sales JM. Long-acting reversible contraception and condom use among female US high school students: implications for sexually transmitted infection prevention. *JAMA Pediatr.* 2016;170:428-434

3. Paul Poteat V, Russell ST, Dewaele A. Sexual health risk behavior disparities among male and female adolescents using identity and behavior indicators of sexual orientation. *Arch Sex Behav.* 2017;https://doi.ortg/10.1007/s10508-017-1082-6
4. Schick VR, Baldwin A, Bay-Cheng LY, Dodge B, Van Der Pol B, Fortenberry JD. "First, I... then, we...": exploring the sequence of sexual acts and safety strategies reported during a sexual encounter using a modified timeline followback method. *Sex Transm Infect.* 2016;92:272-275
5. Richters J, Visser R, Rissel C, Smith A. Sexual practices at last heterosexual encounter and occurrence of orgasm in a national survey. *J Sex Res.* 2006;43:217-226
6. Martinez GM, Abma JC. Sexual activity, contraceptive use, and childbearing of teenagers aged 15-19 in the United States. *NCHS Data Brief.* 2015;209:1-8
7. Manlove J, Ikramullah E, Terry-Humen E. Condom use and consistency among male adolescents in the United States. *J Adolesc Health.* 2008;43:325-333
8. Fortenberry JD, Schick V, Herbenick D, Sanders SA, Dodge B, Reece M. Sexual behaviors and condom use at last vaginal intercourse: a national sample of adolescents ages 14 to 17 years. *J Sex Med.* 2010;7(Suppl 5):305-314
9. Aholou TM, McCree DH, Oraka E, et al. Sexual risk and protective behaviors among reproductive-aged women in the United States. *J Womens Health.* 2017;26:1150-1160
10. Shafii T, Stovel K, Holmes K. Association between condom use at sexual debut and subsequent sexual trajectories: a longitudinal study using biomarkers. *Am J Public Health.* 2007;97:1090-1095
11. Kann L, McManus T, Harris WA, et al. Youth Risk Behavior Surveillance—United States, 2017. *MMWR Surveill Summ.* 2018;67(8):1-114
12. Martinez G, Copen CE, Abma JC. Teenagers in the United States: sexual activity, contraceptive use, and childbearing, 2006-2010 national survey of family growth. *Vital Health Stat 23.* 2011; 31:1-35
13. Williams RL, Fortenberry JD. Update on adolescent condom use. *Curr Opin Obstet Gynecol.* 2011;23:350-354
14. Tyler CP, Whiteman MK, Kraft JM, et al. Dual use of condoms with other contraceptive methods among adolescents and young women in the United States. *J Adolesc Health.* 2014;54:169-175
15. Thompson EL, Vamos CA, Griner SB, Logan R, Vazquez-Otero C, Daley EM. Sexually transmitted infection prevention with long-acting reversible contraception: factors associated with dual use. *Sex Transm Dis.* 2017;44:423-427
16. Struckman-Johnson C, Nalan-Sheffield K, Gaster S, Struckman-Johnson D. Sexual behavior in parked cars reported by Midwestern college men and women. *J Sex Res.* 2017;54:1064-1076
17. Brüll P, Kessels LTE, Repetto L, Dirkson A, Ruiter RAC. ERPs reveal disengagement processes related to condom use embarrassment in intention-behavior inconsistent young adults. *Arch Sex Behav.* 2018;https://doi.org/10.1007/s10508-018-1217-4
18. Shacham E, J Nelson E, Schulte L, Bloomfield M, Murphy R. Geographic variation in condom availability and accessibility. *AIDS Behav.* 2016;20(12):2863-2872
19. Society for Adolescent Health and Medicine. Condom availability in schools: a practical approach to the prevention of sexually transmitted infection/HIV and unintended pregnancy. *J Adolesc Health.* 2017;60:754-757
20. Sadler S, Tosh J, Pennington R, et al. A cost-effectiveness analysis of condom distribution programmes for the prevention of sexually transmitted infections in England. *J Epidemiol Community Health.* 2017;71:897-904
21. Malekinejad M, Parriott A, Blodgett JC, et al. Effectiveness of community-based condom distribution interventions to prevent HIV in the United States: a systematic review and meta-analysis. *PLoS One.* 2017;12(8):e0180718
22. Stover J, Rosen JE, Carvalho MN, et al. The case for investing in the male condom. *PLoS One.* 2017;12(5):e0177108
23. Stover J, Rosen J, Kasedde S, Idele P, McClure C. The impact and cost of the HIV/AIDS investment framework for adolescents. *J Acquir Immune Defic Syndr.* 2014;66:S170-S175
24. Rose E, Diclemente RJ, Wingood GM, et al. The validity of teens' and young adults' self-reported condom use. *Arch Pediatr Adolesc Med.* 2009;163:61-64

25. Kelley CF, Kraft CS, de Man TJ, et al. The rectal mucosa and condomless receptive anal intercourse in HIV-negative MSM: implications for HIV transmission and prevention. *Mucosal Immunol.* 2017;10:996-1007
26. Munk AC, Gudlaugsson E, Malpica A, et al. Consistent condom use increases the regression rate of cervical intraepithelial neoplasia 2-3. *PLoS One.* 2012;7(9):e45114
27. Brown DR, Shew ML, Qadadri B, et al. A longitudinal study of genital human papillomavirus infection in a cohort of closely followed adolescent women. *J Infect Dis.* 2005;191:182-192
28. Shew ML, Fortenberry JD, Tu W, et al. Association of condom use, sexual behaviors, and sexually transmitted infections with the duration of genital human papillomavirus infection among adolescent women. *Arch Pediatr Adolesc Med.* 2006;160:151-156
29. Burchell AN, Tellier PP, Hanley J, Coutlee F, Franco EL. Influence of partner's infection status on prevalent human papillomavirus among persons with a new sex partner. *Sex Transm Dis.* 2010;37(1):34-40
30. Weaver B, Shew M, Qadadri B, et al. Low-level persistence of human papillomavirus 16 DNA in a cohort of closely followed adolescent women. *J Med Virol.* 2011;83:1362-1369
31. Weaver B, Shew M, Qadadri B, et al. Natural history of multiple human papillomavirus infections in female adolescents with prolonged follow-up. *J Adolesc Health.* 2011;48:473-480
32. Mowlabocus S, Harbottle J, Witzel C. What we can't see? Understanding the representations and meanings of UAI, barebacking, and semen exchange in gay male pornography. *J Homosex.* 2014;61:1462-1480
33. Prestage G, Hurley M, Brown G. "Cum play" among gay men. *Arch Sex Behav.* 2013;42:1347-1356
34. Rosenberger JG, Reece M, Schick V, et al. Sexual behaviors and situational characteristics of most recent male-partnered sexual event among gay and bisexually identified men in the United States. *J Sex Med.* 2011;8:3040-3050
35. Hensel DJ, Selby S, Tanner AE, Fortenberry JD. A daily diary analysis of condom breakage and slippage during vaginal sex or anal sex among adolescent women. *Sex Transm Dis.* 2016;43: 531-536
36. Crosby RP, Mena L, Yarber WL, Graham CA, Sanders SA, Milhausen RR. Condom use errors and problems: a comparative study of HIV-positive versus HIV-negative young black men who have sex with men. *Sex Transm Dis.* 2015;42:634-636
37. Crosby RA, Milhausen RR, Mark KP, Yarber WL, Sanders SA, Graham CA. Understanding problems with condom fit and feel: an important opportunity for improving clinic-based safer sex programs. *J Prim Prev.* 2013;34:109-115
38. Levin RJ. Exceptionalism is not exceptional in relation to sexual and reproduction mechanisms: contrasts of human and animal sexuality. *Clin Anat.* 2017;30:940-945
39. Grov C, Wells BE, Parsons JT. Self-reported penis size and experiences with condoms among gay and bisexual men. *Arch Sex Behav.* 2013;42:313-322
40. Grov C, Parsons JT, Bimbi DS. The association between penis size and sexual health among men who have sex with men. *Arch Sex Behav.* 2010;39:788-797
41. Reece M, Briggs L, Dodge B, Herbenick D, Glover R. Perceptions of condom fit and feel among men living with HIV. *AIDS Patient Care STDS.* 2010;24:435-440
42. Soydan H, Akyol İ, Ates F, Yilmaz O, Dursun F, Baykal K. Cross-sectional analysis of penile length in males 13 to 15 years old according to pubertal development stages. *J Urol.* 2012;188:1319-1323
43. Largo RH, Prader A. Pubertal development in Swiss boys. *Helv Paediatr Acta.* 1983;38:211-228
44. Crosby R, Sanders SA, Yarber WL, Graham CA. Condom-use errors and problems: a neglected aspect of studies assessing condom effectiveness. *Am J Prev Med.* 2003;24:367-370
45. Graham CA, Crosby R, Yarber WL, et al. Erection loss in association with condom use among young men attending a public STI clinic: potential correlates and implications for risk behaviour. *Sex Health.* 2006;3(4):255-260
46. Hatherall B, Ingham R, Stone N, McEachran J. How, not just if, condoms are used: the timing of condom application and removal during vaginal sex among young people in England. *Sex Transm Infect.* 2007;83:68-70

47. Sanders SA, Yarber WL, Kaufman EL, Crosby RA, Graham CA, Milhausen RR. Condom use errors and problems: a global view. *Sex Health.* 2012;9:81-95
48. Paz-Bailey G, Koumans EH, Sternberg M, et al. The effect of correct and consistent condom use on chlamydial and gonococcal infection among urban adolescents. *Arch Pediatr Adolesc Med.* 2005;159:536-542
49. Mustanski B, Ryan DT, Garofalo R. Associations of sexually transmitted infections with condom problems among young men who have sex with men. *Sex Transm Dis.* 2014;41:427-432
50. Warner L, Newman DR, Kamb ML, et al; Project RESPECT Study Group. Problems with condom use among patients attending sexually transmitted disease clinics: prevalence, predictors, and relation to incident gonorrhea and chlamydia. *Am J Epidemiol.* 2008;167:341-349
51. Yarber WL, Milhausen RR, Beavers KA, et al. A pilot test of a self-guided, home-based intervention to improve condom-related sexual experiences, attitudes, and behaviors among young women. *J Am Coll Health.* 2018;66:421-428
52. Shepherd LM, Sly KF, Girard JM. Comparison of comprehensive and abstinence-only sexuality education in young African American adolescents. *J Adolesc.* 2017;61:50-63
53. Matson PA, Fortenberry JD, Chung S-e, Gaydos CA, Ellen JM. Weekly variations in feelings of trust predict incident STI within a prospective cohort of adolescent women from a US city. *Sex Transm Infect.* 2018;doi:10.1136/sextrans-2017-053431
54. Bird JDP, Eversman M, Voisin DR. 'You just can't trust everybody': the impact of sexual risk, partner type and perceived partner trustworthiness on HIV-status disclosure decisions among HIV-positive black gay and bisexual men. *Cult Health Sex.* 2017;19:829-843
55. Norona JC, Welsh DP, Olmstead SB, Bliton CF. The symbolic nature of trust in heterosexual adolescent romantic relationships. *Arch Sex Behav.* 2017;46:1673-1684
56. Watkins SJ, Boon SD. Expectations regarding partner fidelity in dating relationships. *J Soc Pers Rel.* 2016;33:237-256
57. Mullinax M, Sanders S, Higgins J, Dennis B, Reece M, Fortenberry JD. Establishment of safety paradigms and trust in emerging adult relationships. *Cult Health Sex.* 2016;18:890-904
58. Feldstein Ewing SW, Bryan AD. A question of love and trust? The role of relationship factors in adolescent sexual decision making. *J Dev Behav Pediatr.* 2015;36:628-634
59. Towner SL, Dolcini MM, Harper GW. Romantic relationship dynamics of urban African American adolescents: patterns of monogamy, commitment, and trust. *Youth Soc.* 2015;47:343-373
60. Harvey SM, Washburn I, Oakley L, Warren J, Sanchez D. Competing priorities: partner-specific relationship characteristics and motives for condom use among at-risk young adults. *J Sex Res.* 2017;54:665-676
61. Milhausen RR, McKay A, Graham CA, et al. Do associations between pleasure ratings and condom use during penile–vaginal intercourse vary by relationship type?: a study of Canadian university students. *J Sex Res.* 2018;55:21-30
62. Senn TE, Scott-Sheldon LA, Carey MP. Relationship-specific condom attitudes predict condom use among STD clinic patients with both primary and non-primary partners. *AIDS Behav.* 2014;18:1420-1427
63. Calabrese SK, Reisen CA, Zea MC, Poppen PJ, Bianchi FT. The pleasure principle: the effect of perceived pleasure loss associated with condoms on unprotected anal intercourse among immigrant Latino men who have sex with men. *AIDS Patient Care STDS.* 2012;26:430-435
64. Rosenberger JG, Bell DL, McBride KR, Fortenberry JD, Ott MA. Condoms and developmental contexts in younger adolescent boys. *Sex Transm Infect.* 2010;86:400-403
65. Crosby RA, Mena L. Correlates of enhanced sexual pleasure from condom use: a study of young black men who have sex with men in the United States. *AIDS Behav.* 2017;21:1491-1496
66. Hensel DJ, Stupiansky NW, Herbenick D, Dodge B, Reece M. Sexual pleasure during condom-protected vaginal sex among heterosexual men. *J Sex Med.* 2012;9:1272-1276
67. Wolfs K, Bos AER, Mevissen FEF, Peters G-JY, van Lankveld JJDM. Sexual arousal and implicit and explicit determinants of condom use intentions. *Arch Sex Behav.* 2018;doi:10.1007/s10508-018-1257-9

68. Khurana A, Romer D, Betancourt LM, Brodsky NL, Giannetta JM, Hurt H. Stronger working memory reduces sexual risk taking in adolescents, even after controlling for parental influences. *Child Dev.* 2015;86:1125-1141
69. Epperson CN, Amin Z, Ruparel K, Gur R, Loughead J. Interactive effects of estrogen and serotonin on brain activation during working memory and affective processing in menopausal women. *Psychoneuroendocrinology.* 2012;37:372-382
70. Spronk M, Jonkman LM. Electrophysiological evidence for different effects of working memory load on interference control in adolescents than adults. *Int J Psychophysiol.* 2012;83:24-35
71. Malagoli C, Usai MC. The effects of gender and age on inhibition and working memory organization in 14- to 19-year-old adolescents and young adults. *Cogn Devel.* 2018;45:10-23
72. O'Sullivan LF, Brotto LA, Byers ES, Majerovich JA, Wuest JA. Prevalence and characteristics of sexual functioning among sexually experienced middle to late adolescents. *J Sex Med.* 2014;11: 630-641
73. Akre C, Berchtold A, Gmel G, Suris J-C. The evolution of sexual dysfunction in young men aged 18–25 years. *J Adolesc Health.* 2014;55:736-743
74. Apodaca TR, Moser NC. The use and abuse of prescription medication to facilitate or enhance sexual behavior among adolescents. *Clin Pharmacol Ther.* 2011;89:22-24
75. Lin X, Mattson CL, Freedman M, Skarbinski J; Medical Monitoring Project. Erectile dysfunction medication prescription and condomless intercourse in HIV-infected men who have sex with men in the United States. *AIDS Behav.* 2017;21:1129-1137
76. Graham CA, Crosby R, Sanders S, Milhausen R, Yarber WL. Condom-associated erection problems: a study of high-risk young black males residing in the southern United States. *Am J Mens Health.* 2016;10:141-145
77. Elmerstig E, Thomten J. Vulvar pain-associations between first-time vaginal intercourse, tampon insertion, and later experiences of pain. *J Sex Marital Ther.* 2016;42:707-720
78. Herbenick D, Schick V, Sanders SA, Reece M, Fortenberry JD. Pain experienced during vaginal and anal intercourse with other-sex partners: findings from a nationally representative probability study in the United States. *J Sex Med.* 2015;12:1040-1051
79. De Rosa CJ, Ethier KA, Kim DH, et al. Sexual intercourse and oral sex among public middle school students: prevalence and correlates. *Perspect Sex Reprod Health.* 2010;42:197-205
80. Habel MA, Leichliter JS, Dittus PJ, Spicknall IH, Aral SO. Heterosexual anal and oral sex in adolescents and adults in the United States, 2011-2015. *Sex Transm Dis.* 2018;doi:10.1097/olq.0000000000000889
81. Glynn TR, Operario D, Montgomery M, Almonte A, Chan PA. The duality of oral sex for men who have sex with men: an examination into the increase of sexually transmitted infections amid the age of HIV prevention. *AIDS Patient Care STD.* 2017;31:261-267
82. Stone N, Hatherall B, Ingham R, McEachran J. Oral sex and condom use among young people in the United Kingdom. *Perspect Sex Reprod Health.* 2006;38:6-12
83. Hui B, Fairley CK, Chen M, et al. Oral and anal sex are key to sustaining gonorrhoea at endemic levels in MSM populations: a mathematical model. *Sex Transm Infect.* 2015;91:365-369
84. Remez L. Oral sex among adolescents: is it sex or is it abstinence? *Fam Plann Perspect.* 2000;32: 298-304
85. Fava NM, Bay-Cheng LY. Young women's adolescent experiences of oral sex: relation of age of initiation to sexual motivation, sexual coercion, and psychological functioning. *J Adolesc.* 2012;35:1191-1201
86. Bay-Cheng LY, Robinson AD, Zucker AN. Behavioral and relational contexts of adolescent desire, wanting, and pleasure: undergraduate women's retrospective accounts. *J Sex Res.* 2009;46:511-524
87. Hensel DJ, Fortenberry JD, Orr DP. Variations in coital and noncoital sexual repertoire among adolescent women. *J Adolesc Health.* 2008;42:170-176
88. Hess KL, Crepaz N, Rose C, Purcell D, Paz-Bailey G. Trends in sexual behavior among men who have sex with men (MSM) in high-income countries, 1990-2013: a systematic review. *AIDS Behav.* 2017;21:2811-2834

89. Kapadia F, Bub K, Barton S, Stults CB, Halkitis PN. Longitudinal trends in sexual behaviors without a condom among sexual minority youth: the P18 Cohort Study. *AIDS Behav.* 2015;19: 2152-2161
90. Molina JM, Charreau I, Spire B, et al. Efficacy, safety, and effect on sexual behaviour of on-demand pre-exposure prophylaxis for HIV in men who have sex with men: an observational cohort study. *Lancet HIV.* 2017;4:e402-e410
91. Greene GJ, Andrews R, Kuper L, Mustanski B. Intimacy, monogamy, and condom problems drive unprotected sex among young men in serious relationships with other men: a mixed methods dyadic study. *Arch Sex Behav.* 2014;43:73-87
92. Newcomb M, Mustanski B. Developmental change in the effects of sexual partner and relationship characteristics on sexual risk behavior in young men who have sex with men. *AIDS Behav.* 2016;20(6):1284-1294
93. Ybarra ML, Prescott TL, Phillips GL 2nd, Bull SS, Parsons JT, Mustanski B. Pilot RCT results of an mHealth HIV prevention program for sexual minority male adolescents. *Pediatrics.* 2017;140(1):e20162999
94. Oidtman J, Sherman SG, Morgan A, German D, Arrington-Sanders R. Satisfaction and condomless anal sex at sexual debut and sexual risk among young black same-sex attracted men. *Arch Sex Behav.* 2017;46:947-959
95. Roth EA, Cui Z, Rich A, et al. Seroadaptive strategies of Vancouver gay and bisexual men in a treatment as prevention environment. *J Homosex.* 2018;65:524-539
96. Purcell DW, Higa D, Mizuno Y, Lyles C. Quantifying the harms and benefits from serosorting among HIV-negative gay and bisexual men: a systematic review and meta-analysis. *AIDS Behav.* 2017;21:2835-2843
97. Paz-Bailey G, Mendoza MC, Finlayson T, et al; NHBS Study Group. Trends in condom use among MSM in the United States: the role of antiretroviral therapy and seroadaptive strategies. *AIDS.* 2016;30:1985-1990
98. Khosropour CM, Dombrowski JC, Swanson F, et al. Trends in serosorting and the association with HIV/STI risk over time among men who have sex with men. *J Acquir Immune Defic Syndr.* 2016;72:189-197
99. Remis RS, Alary M, Liu J, Kaul R, Palmer RW. HIV transmission among men who have sex with men due to condom failure. *PLoS One.* 2014;9(9):e107540
100. Rodriguez K, Ventura-DiPersia C, LeVasseur MT, Kelvin EA. Inconsistencies on U.S. Departments of Health websites regarding anal use of the female condom. *AIDS Behav.* 2015;19: 1141-1149
101. Mantell JE, Kelvin EA, Exner TM, Hoffman S, Needham S, Stein ZA. Anal use of the female condom: does uncertainty justify provider inaction? *AIDS Care.* 2009;21:1185-1194
102. Kelvin EA, Mantell JE, Candelario N, et al. Off-label use of the female condom for anal intercourse among men in New York City. *Am J Public Health.* 2011;101:2241-2244
103. Beksinska M, Greener R, Kleinschmidt I, Pillay L, Maphumulo V, Smit J. A randomized noninferiority crossover controlled trial of the functional performance and safety of new female condoms: an evaluation of the Velvet, Cupid2, and FC2. *Contraception.* 2015;92:261-267
104. Weeks MR, Zhan W, Li J, Hilario H, Abbott M, Medina Z. Female condom use and adoption among men and women in a general low-income urban U.S. population. *AIDS Behav.* 2015;19: 1642-1654
105. Holtgrave DR, Maulsby C, Kharfen M, et al. Cost-utility analysis of a female condom promotion program in Washington, DC. *AIDS Behav.* 2012;16:1115-1120
106. Witte SS, MacPhee C, Ginsburg N, Deshmukh N. Medicaid reimbursement for the female condom. *Am J Public Health.* 2017;107:1633-1635
107. Maksut JL, Eaton LA. Female condoms = missed opportunities: lessons learned from promotion-centered interventions. *Womens Health Issues.* 2015;25:366-376
108. Beksinska M, Smit J, Greener R, Piaggio G, Joanis C. The female condom learning curve: patterns of female condom failure over 20 uses. *Contraception.* 2015;91:85-90

109. Richters J, Clayton S. The practical and symbolic purpose of dental dams in lesbian safer sex promotion. *Sex Health.* 2010;7:103-106
110. Ybarra ML, Rosario M, Saewyc E, Goodenow C. Sexual behaviors and partner characteristics by sexual identity among adolescent girls. *J Adolesc Health.* 2016;58:310-316
111. Yap L, Richters J, Butler T, Schneider K, Kirkwood K, Donovan B. Sexual practices and dental dam use among women prisoners—a mixed methods study. *Sex Health.* 2010;7:170-176
112. Richters J, Prestage G, Schneider K, Clayton S. Do women use dental dams? Safer sex practices of lesbians and other women who have sex with women. *Sex Health.* 2010;7:165-169
113. Muzny CA, Harbison HS, Pembleton ES, Hook EW, Austin EL. Misperceptions regarding protective barrier method use for safer sex among African-American women who have sex with women. *Sex Health.* 2013;10:138-141

Adolesc Med 030 (2019) 60–81

The Contraceptive Ring, Patch, and Pills: An Update

Sophia Yen, MD, MPH[a*]; Erica P. Cahill, MD[b]

[a]*Division of Adolescent Medicine, Department of Pediatrics, Stanford Medical School, Palo Alto, California;* [b]*Department of Obstetrics and Gynecology, Stanford Medical School, Palo Alto, California*

LEARNING OBJECTIVES

After reviewing this article, the reader should be able to:

1. Counsel patients on the differences between the contraceptive ring, patch, and pill
2. Manage common adverse effects from combined hormonal contraceptives (CHCs), such as breakthrough bleeding and nausea
3. Cite 3 non-contraceptive benefits of CHC

INTRODUCTION

Access to effective contraception is one of the pillars of adolescent health. Besides preventing pregnancy, hormonal contraceptives are an important tool for treating a variety of common medical problems among adolescents such as acne, polycystic ovary syndrome, and dysmenorrhea.

Sexual intercourse is common among adolescents, with recent data showing that among 15- to 19-year-olds, 44% of young women and 49% of young men have had sexual intercourse; these rates have been relatively unchanged since 2002. From 2006 to 2010, 86% of females and 93% of males aged 15 to 19 years reported having used contraceptives the last time they had sex.[1]

---

*Corresponding author
E-mail address: sophia@pandiahealth.com

 ISSN 1934-4287

Teenage pregnancy is an immense public health problem in the United States, with teenagers aged 15 to 19 years accounting for more than 200,000 births in 2016, approximately 5.3% of all births in the United States.[1] A pregnancy during adolescence can have lasting health, economic, and social implications for the teenager, her potential child, and society. Teenage pregnancy rates have been decreasing over the past few years to a rate of 20 per 1000 births as a result of improved access to contraception, including long-acting reversible contraception (LARC) such as intrauterine devices (IUDs) and contraceptive implants.[2,3] However, this rate remains substantially higher than those in other developed countries.[4] Although research about adolescents and LARC use has shown a 70% acceptance rate when given easy access, many adolescents continue to choose short-acting hormonal contraceptive options.[5] Because of myths regarding who is a good candidate for LARC, limited access to LARC providers, cost, and the beneficial non-contraceptive effects and ease of access for teenagers, short-acting combined hormonal contraceptives (CHCs) are often the first medical methods accessed by female teenagers. This review summarizes the current options for short-acting CHCs for adolescents and their use, benefits, risks, non-contraceptive uses, and areas for further research.

CONTRACEPTIVE COUNSELING

Before the provision of contraceptives, it is important to be reasonably certain that a woman is not currently pregnant. The Centers for Disease Control and Prevention (CDC) has provided guidelines for ensuring a woman is unlikely to be pregnant.[6] These guidelines allow physicians to offer convenient contraception options to women rather than having them wait to prove that they are not pregnant. For same-day start, women should meet at least one of the following criteria: less than 7 days after the start of normal menses, have not had vaginal intercourse since last normal menses, have been consistently using a reliable method of contraception, is within 4 weeks postpartum, is fully or almost fully breastfeeding *and* amenorrheic *and* are less than 6 months postpartum, or are less than 7 days from an induced or spontaneous abortion.[6] However, when a physician is uncertain whether the woman might be pregnant, the benefits of starting the implant, depot medroxyprogesterone acetate (DMPA), CHCs, and progestin-only pills (POPs) likely exceed any risk; therefore, starting the method should be considered at any time, with a follow-up pregnancy test in 2 to 4 weeks.

After the Contraceptive CHOICE project,[5] a new paradigm shift in contraceptive counseling has taken place, emphasizing LARC including IUDs and contraceptive implants as the best first-choice option and moving to more user-dependent options if patients are not interested in LARC.[7] However, not all patients, particularly teenagers, are ready or interested in these options because of the invasive nature. Additionally, research and the Reproductive Justice movement have shown increased recommendation of long-acting methods to specific groups of historically disempowered women, including women of color and

Table 1
Contraception ever use 2011-2015: sexually experienced women aged 15 to 19 years

Method	%
Condom	97
Withdrawal	60
Pill	56
Emergency contraception	23
Depo-Provera	17
Fertility awareness	12
Ring	5
Intrauterine device	3
Implant	3
Patch	2

Data from Abma JC, Martinez, GM. Sexual activity and contraceptive use among teenagers in the United States, 2011-2015. *Natl Health Stat Report*. 2017;104:1-23.

low-income women.[8] Studies demonstrate that even with increased knowledge of and access to LARC, combined hormonal methods are still the most common group of contraceptives among adolescents (Table 1).[9] This may be the result of ease of access, lack of need for pelvic examinations, or their non-contraceptive benefits, particularly acne treatment.

When discussing the efficacy of contraceptive methods, physicians should know the difference between *perfect use* (data that come from clinical trials) and *typical use* (based on survey data of failure rates in 1 year of use) (Table 2). Particularly with CHC methods for which efficacy depends on regular and appropriate use, counseling patients on the logistics of best use and what to do in the case of imperfect use are important for maximizing efficacy. Physicians should also understand the CDC U.S. Medical Eligibility Criteria (US MEC) for Contraceptive Use, which have a numerical risk-to-benefit score for clinical conditions for each type of contraception.[10] The scores range from 1 (without restrictions) to 4 (an unacceptable health risk if the contraceptive method is used). The clinician and the patient together should weigh the risks of any contraceptive method use against the risks of unintended pregnancy.

Before starting any prescription contraception, a complete medical history and blood pressure measurement should be obtained. Of note for telemedicine practices, per the CDC guidelines, "if access to health care is limited" the blood pressure can be obtained "in non-clinical settings such as pharmacies or fire stations" and reported to her provider.[6]

Table 2
Contraceptive efficacy: typical versus perfect

Method	Women experiencing unintended pregnancy (%) in first year of use		
	Typical use[a]	Perfect use[a]	Continue at 1 year (%)
No method	85	85	—
Withdrawal	28	18	46
Condom (male)	18	2	43
Combined oral contraceptive pill	7	0.3	55[b]
Patch	7	0.3	49[b]
Ring	7	0.3	54[b]

[a] Hatcher RA, Nelson AI, Trussell J, et al, eds. *Contraceptive Technology.* 21st ed. New York, NY: Ayer Company Publishers, Inc; 2018, with permission.
[b] Peipert JF, Zhao Q, Allsworth JE, et al. Continuation and satisfaction of reversible contraception. *Obstet Gynecol.* 2011;117(5):1105-1113, with permission.

SHORT-ACTING CHC METHODS

Overview

Mechanism of Action

The mechanism of action for CHCs has not changed over the years and is the same for the ring, patch, and combined oral contraceptive pill (OCP). Estrogen and progestin mimic a luteal phase and inhibit ovulation through negative feedback on the hypothalamic-pituitary-ovarian axis, suppressing follicle-stimulating hormone and the luteinizing hormone surge. Progestin thins the lining of the endometrium, making it inhospitable for implantation. Progestin also thickens the cervical mucus (increasing the difficulty for sperm to enter the uterus) and decreases the motility of the cilia in the fallopian tubes. Progestin-only pills function mainly through cervical mucus changes and less reliably inhibit ovulation.

Differences in Progestins

Synthetic progestins are divided into 3 families and 4 generations: estranes (first-generation), gonanes (includes: second- and third-generation), and drospirenone (fourth generation). Estranes include ethynodiol, norethindrone, and norethindrone acetate. Estranes convert to the biologically active norethindrone. Estranes have shorter half-lives (8 hours vs 16 hours). In comparison, gonanes are more potent. Gonanes include norgestrel, levonorgestrel (LNG), desogestrel, norgestimate, gestodene, and dienogest. Levonorgestrel is the prototypical gonane and the active isomer of norgestrel. It has less individual variability because it does not undergo first-pass metabolism compared to norethindrone. See Tables 3 and 4 for comparison of the various progestins' and CHC OCPs' androgenic versus progestational potency.

In the 1980s, 3 high-potency gonanes with lower androgenic adverse effects were developed: norgestimate, desogestrel, and gestodene. Norgestimate has the lowest androgen receptor binding affinity and LNG has the highest. Norgestimate and desogestrel increase sex hormone binding globulin, which results in lower circulating testosterone.

Drosperinone is an analogue of spironolactone and is roughly equivalent to 25 mg of spironolactone in its antimineralocorticoid effects. In 2012, the FDA issued a drug safety communication stating "drospirenone-containing birth control pills may be associated with a higher risk for blood clots than other progestin-containing pills" and cited evidence that some epidemiologic studies showed a 3-fold increase in risk and some studies showed no increase in risk. Drosperinone is contraindicated for patients at risk for hyperkalemia (renal disease), hepatic dysfunction, and adrenal insufficiency. Its diuretic effect may exacerbate headaches in people who are prone to them by inducing a relative dehydration state.

Vaginal Ring

The contraceptive vaginal ring (NuvaRing; Merck, Organon) is a plastic (ethylene vinyl) ring that releases a combination of estrogen/progestin daily (15 mcg ethinyl estradiol [EE], 120 mcg etonogestrel). Etonogestrel is the active

Table 3
Progestin potency

Progestin Type (1 mg)	**Progestational Activity (relative to 1 mg of norethindrone)**	**Androgenic Activity (relative to 1 mg of norethindrone)**
norethindrone	1	1
norethindrone acetate	1.2	1.6
ethynodiol diacetate	1.4	0.6
levonorgestrel	5.3	8.3
dl-norgestrel	2.6	4.2
norgestimate	1.3	1.9
norelgestromin	1.3	1.9
desogestrel	9	3.4
drospirenone	1.5	0

Reproduced with permission from Dickey RP. *Managing Contraceptive Pill Patients*. 15th ed. Fort Collins, CO; EMIS Inc. Medical Publishers; 2014.

Table 4
Progestins (from least androgenic to most androgenic) and Progestational Activity

Progestin Type	Androgenic activity	Progestin (mg)	Progestational activity	mcg EE	Brand names
Drosperinone	0.00	3.00	4.50	20	Gianvi, Loryna, Nikki, Vestura, Yaz
Drosperinone	0.00	3.00	4.50	30	Ocella, Syeda, Yasmin, Zarah
Norelgestromin	0.29	0.15	0.20	20	Xulane
Norethindrone	0.40	0.40	0.40	35	Balzivia, Briellyn, Gildagia, Ovcon 35, Philith, Zenchent
Etonogestrel*	0.41	0.12	1.08	15	NuvaRing
Norgestimate	0.48	0.25	0.33	35	Ortho-Cyclen
Norethindrone	0.50	0.50	0.50	35	Brevicon, Modicon, Necon 0.5/35, Nelova 0.5/35, NEE 0.5/35
Norethindrone	0.50	0.50	0.50	35	Ortho-Novum, Jenest, Necon 10/11, NEE 10.11
Desogestrel	0.51	0.15	1.35	20	Kariva, Mircette, Kimidess, Pimtrea, Viorele
Desogestrel	0.51	0.15	1.35	30	Apri, Desogen, Emoquette, Enskyce, Ortho-Cept, Reclipsen
Ethynodiol diacetate	0.60	1.00	1.40	35	Demulen, Zovia, Kelnor
Levonorgestrel	0.83	0.10	0.53	20	Aviane, Levlite, Lutera, Alesse
Norethindrone	1.00	1.00	1.00	20/30/35	Estrostep Fe, Tilia, Tri-Legest
Norethindrone	1.00	1.00	1.00	35	Cyclafem, Dasetta, Necon 1/35, Nelova 1/35, NEE 1/35, Genora 1/35, Norcept-E 1/35, Norethin 1/35E, Norinyl 1/35, Ortho-Novum 1/35
Norethindrone	1.00	1.00	1.00	50	Necon 1/50, Norinyl 1/50, Ortho-Novum 1/50, Ovcon 50
Levonorgestrel	1.25	0.15	0.80	30	Chateal, Jolessa, Levlen, Levora, Nordette, Portia, Seasonale, Seasonique
Norgestrel	1.26	0.30	0.78	30	Lo Ovral, Low Ogestrel
Norethindrone acetate	1.60	1.00	1.20	20	Blisovi, Gildess, Junel 1/20, Larin, Loestrin 1/20, Microgestin 1/20
Norethindrone acetate	2.40	1.50	1.80	30	Blisovi, Gildess, Junel 1.5/30, Larin, Loestrin 1.5/30, Microgestin 1.5/30

EE, ethinyl estradiol.
* Etonogestrel assumed to be equivalent to desogestrel.
Data derived from GoodRx Web site https://www.goodrx.com/ and Jelovsek FR. Which Oral Contraceptive is Best for Me? Women's Health Web Site. https://www.wdxcyber.com/ncontr13.htm. Accessed November 27, 2018.

metabolite of desogestrel. The vaginal ring is a soft, flexible ring that measures 54 mm in diameter and 4 mm in thickness. It is inserted into the vagina and sits around the cervix. Each ring is dosed for efficacy for up to 35 days, but typically a new ring is left in place for 3 weeks then removed for up to 7 days for withdrawal bleed. Young women should be instructed to insert a new ring within 7 days even if bleeding continues. Continuous use of the vaginal ring for up to 35 days at a time is also an option without a change in efficacy, although women may experience increased vaginal spotting with continuous use.[11] The ring can be removed for up to 3 hours at a time without effect on efficacy.[12] Similar to other hormonal contraceptive methods, the schedule of when and how often the patient bleeds can be individualized by the patient. The NuvaRing can be stored for up to 4 months at room temperature (between 59 and 86°F). Avoid direct sunlight or storing above 86°F.[12]

Efficacy and Safety Concerns

The pregnancy rate is 0.65 per 100 woman-years. Adherence with the vaginal ring is higher than with OCPs: 90.8% versus 78% of women reported using it reliably.[9,13] Many young women are concerned about the risk of expulsion, which is rare but can occur. Expulsion usually is related to constipation, tampon removal, or intercourse. A study evaluating whether the ring could be expelled with Valsalva maneuver found that among 80 young women, none were able to expel the ring.[14]

Research has shown that use of the contraceptive vaginal ring has minimal effects on lipid levels, glucose metabolism, or blood pressure. Minimal effect on hemostatic variables compared with 30 mcg EE and 150 mcg LNG also has been reported.[15] Thrombogenic markers improve in women switching from CHC pills to the ring, suggesting a reduced risk of venous thromboembolism (VTE) in women who changed to the ring. Low androgenic effects were confirmed with elevated sex hormone binding globulin levels.[16] Contraceptive efficacy is not changed when the contraceptive ring is used with antimycotic medications, tampons, or spermicide.[17,18]

Counseling Considerations

Adolescents interested in this method should feel comfortable inserting and removing the ring. Ideally, the ring remains in place during sexual intercourse but can be removed for up to 3 hours.

New Options on the Horizon

A new 1-year vaginal ring was approved by the US Food and Drug Administration (FDA) in August 2018, creating the first long-acting option that is under a woman's direct control.[19] The new vaginal contraceptive ring (Annovera; Population Council) is made of silicone elastomer and contains 103 mg segesterone acetate and 17.4 mg EE, releasing on average 0.15 mg/day segesterone acetate and 0.013 mg/day EE.[20] Patients are instructed to insert the ring for 21 days continuously and then remove it for a 7-day interval, similar to the currently available NuvaRing. The ring can then be cleaned and reinserted, without additional prescriptions. The Annovera provides enough medication for thirteen 28-day cycles or 1 year of use. The 1-year contraceptive vaginal ring does not require refrigeration, which will be particularly important in low-resource areas. The package insert instructs users to remove the ring for no more than 2 hours at a time to continue efficacy.

The Annovera has a perfect use efficacy rate of 97.3%.[20] However, the trials did not include women with body mass index (BMI) greater than 29, and a "limitation of use" statement on the labeling indicates that the efficacy in women with higher BMIs is not known. In addition to the general contraindications to CHCs, other contraindications specific to this ring include use of hepatitis C drugs containing ombitasvir, paritaprevir, or ritonavir. [20]

Additionally, a new vaginal ring containing segesterone acetate and EE for continuous 90-day use is currently under investigation.[21]

Contraceptive Patch

The contraceptive patch (Xulane; Mylan Pharmaceuticals) contains 0.53 mg EE and 4.86 mg norelgestromin, an active metabolite of norgestimate. It releases approximately 150 mcg/day norelgestromin and 35 mcg/day EE. Typically, patches are used for 3 weeks then removed for 5 to 7 days, and a new patch is placed. Alternatively, women can use the contraceptive patch continuously for up to 12 weeks, as daily levels of EE during this time remain within the range of product labeling (0-193 pg/mL).[22] However, given the accumulation of approximately 2.15 pg/mL estradiol per week over the course of 12 weeks, generally continuous use beyond 12 weeks is not encouraged because levels of estradiol and the risk of VTE have not been studied.

Efficacy and Safety Concerns

The typical failure rate is approximately 7%.[23] The annual probability of pregnancy was 0.8% in a review of 3319 women.[24] The only patch available in the United States is Xulane. The Ortho Evra patch, which contained 6 mg norelgestromin and 75 mg of EE, was discontinued in 2014. Research has shown that the contraceptive patch exposes a woman to about 60% more estrogen than the standard 35 mcg EE in CHC pills, leading to a black box warning in 2011 regarding increased risk of blood clots. The contraceptive patch package specifically states that the patch may be less effective in women who weigh more than 98 kg (190 pounds) and may have increased risks of VTE in all women, especially those at higher baseline risk.[25] Counseling of adolescents, particularly obese adolescents, should thoroughly review these factors.

The warning specifically states "The risk of VTE among women aged 15 to 44 who used the norelgestromin and ethinyl estradiol transdermal system compared to women who used several different oral contraceptives was assessed in 5 US epidemiologic studies using electronic healthcare claims data. The relative risk estimates ranged from 1.2 to 2.2; one of the studies found a statistically significant increased relative risk of VTE for current users of norelgestromin and ethinyl estradiol transdermal system."[25]

Women should be instructed to apply the patch directly to the skin, without lotion or other chemicals on the skin. The patch can be applied to the buttock, abdomen, upper outer arm, or upper torso. There are no restrictions on activities while using the patch (eg, women may swim, bathe, and use saunas). Overall the patch rarely becomes detached; however, in 1 study of adolescents, 35% experienced complete or partial detachment over a 3-month period.[26]

It is believed the slightly higher efficacy of the patch compared to CHC pills can be attributed to needing to remember to change a patch once per week instead of remembering to take a pill every day. In 1 trial, women were more likely to correctly use the patch (88%) than correctly use CHCs (78%).[27]

The most common adverse events resulting in discontinuation were skin reactions (1.9%), nausea (1.8%), emotional lability (1.5%), headache (1.1%), and breast discomfort (1.0%).[28] Skin irritation from use of the contraceptive patch has been reported in 20% of women, although this is rarely an allergy. A more common adverse effect with use of the patch versus standard CHC pills is breakthrough bleeding/spotting, which was around 18% for the patch versus 11% for CHC pills for the first 2 cycles. By the third cycle, breakthrough bleeding/spotting was reported in 10% of women using the patch versus 8.8% for women taking CHC pills, and decreased to 5.5% versus 7.1% by month 13.[27] Breast tenderness may be higher because of higher estrogen exposure from the patch compared to standard CHCs.

Pharmacokinetic Profile of Transdermal EE

The pharmacokinetic (PK) profile for the norelgestromin and EE transdermal system is different from the PK profile for oral contraceptives in that it has higher steady-state concentrations of EE and a lower peak concentration. Area under the curve and average concentration at steady state for EE are approximately 60% higher in women using the transdermal system than in women using an oral contraceptive containing 35 mcg EE. In contrast, the peak concentration for EE is approximately 25% lower in women using the transdermal system.[25] Whether the risk of serious adverse events changes based on the differences in PK profiles of EE in women using the norelgestromin and EE transdermal system compared with women using CHC pills containing 30 to 35 mcg EE is not known. Increased estrogen exposure may increase the risk of adverse events, including VTE.

Combined Hormonal Contraceptive Pills

Combined hormonal contraceptive pills are the most common type of contraception used by young women aged 15 to 19 years.[9] The primary mechanism of action is inhibition of ovulation. The progestin component inhibits luteal surge and ovulation, while the estrogen component inhibits follicular development and potentiates the progestin effects. For the prescriber, choosing a pill to start with or changing pill type depends on the desired estrogen level, progestin type, and whether a patient wants monthly cycles or semicontinuous cycling. Prescribers should note that progestin type and dosage determine many of a pill's benefits and adverse effects. The CHC pill should be taken daily, but because of its longer half-life it does not need to be taken at the same time every day.

All combination CHCs contain EE, but the dose ranges from 10 to 50 mcg EE per pill. In general, adolescents and women of bone density accrual age (15-30 years) should be taking a minimum of 30 mcg EE. Scholes et al[29] concluded that less than 30 mcg EE may adversely affect the bone density of young women. Typically, physicians prescribe lower-dose estrogen pills to women who cannot tolerate higher dosages because of nausea.

Many formulations have added some form of iron to the placebo pills, and some have estrogen-only pills in an attempt to decrease bleeding time during the placebo week.

Continuous Use

There is no medical reason for a woman using CHC to have a withdrawal bleed. For a woman not using hormonal contraception, her endogenous progesterone level is high only during the luteal phase of her cycle. Because most hormonal contraception is progestin-based, the continuous progestin exposure results in a thin, decidualized endometrial lining. Research has demonstrated that most women of all income levels prefer to have fewer withdrawal bleeds or no withdrawal bleeding at all.[11,30] Several contraceptive methods can eliminate the monthly bleed, such as the contraceptive shot, implant, and progesterone IUD. Women who have bleeding disorders, endometriosis, or premenstrual dysphoric disorder, for example, may prefer these methods. The disadvantage of continuous or semi-continuous use of hormonal contraception is less predictability in bleeding episodes. In 2003, the first OCP designed to have 3 months of continuous use was introduced (Seasonale: 150 mcg LNG, 30 mcg EE; Teva Pharmaceuticals), followed in 2008 by the first combined OCP to be taken continuously without a week of placebo pills (Lybrel: 90 mcg LNG, 20 mcg EE; Wyeth Pharmaceuticals). Lybrel has since been discontinued. Generic versions of continuous-use pills have become available, and a pill, in which the placebo week is replaced by estrogen-only pills, has come to market as well (Seasonique; 84 tablets of 150 mcg LNG, 30 mcg EE, 7 tablets of 10 mcg EE; Teva Pharmaceuticals). Although these continuous use CHC exist, any CHC pill can be used continuously. Patients can be instructed to skip the placebo week and go straight into the next pack.

Limited Use for Triphasic Pills

Triphasic contraceptive pills were created to mimic a woman's natural cycle. However, this continuous monthly cycling is not natural,[31,32] and women experience fewer adverse effects on a stable level of hormones with various disorders (eg, catamenial seizures and diabetes mellitus).[33] See Table 5. Thus, prescribers should generally avoid prescribing triphasic pills unless there is a need for a specific formulation (eg, 10 mcg EE plus norgestimate) or a 25% to 33% lower progestin over the course of the month.

Table 5
Medical conditions improved by continuous hormonal contraceptive use

Hematologic disorders
Inherited anemia: sickle cell, thalassemia, Fanconi anemia
Inherited bleeding disorders: von Willebrand disease, hemophilia, other factor deficiencies
Anticoagulation
Hematologic or other malignancy: chemotherapy, bone marrow transplantation
Other hematologic conditions: thrombocytopenia, idiopathic thrombocytopenic purpura, afibrinogenemia
Gynecologic conditions
Endometriosis
Premenstrual syndrome/premenstrual dysphoric disorder
Menorrhagia: anemia due to anovulatory bleeding, idiopathic menorrhagia
Dysmenorrhea
Infectious diseases, blood-borne
Human immunodeficiency virus
Hepatitis B, hepatitis C
Developmental disabilities
Moderate-to-severe developmental delay
Cerebral palsy with physical limitation for hygiene
Medical conditions with catamenial exacerbation
Asthma
Arthritis
Depression
Diabetes control
Neurologic disorders
Catamenial seizures
Migraine disorders caused by menses
Non-medical conditions
Quality of life, menstrual cycle timing control
Environmental, using fewer sanitary products
Deployed military personnel

Derived from Altshuler AL, Hillard PJ. Menstrual suppression for adolescents. *Curr Opin Obstet Gynecol.* 2014;26(5):323-331

Progestin-Only Pills

Progestin-only pills work mainly by thickening the cervical mucus, thinning the endometrium, and to a lesser extent by preventing ovulation, because about 40% of women continue to ovulate on POPs.[34] In the United States, POPs all provide only norethindrone, 35 mcg daily. They do not contain estrogen.

Counseling Considerations

It is important to counsel patients that POPs must be taken continuously (ie, no placebo pills) and typically within 3 hours of the same time every day. If a patient is more than 3 hours late taking the POP, she should use emergency contraception (if she had heterosexual vaginal intercourse during that time period) and abstain from intercourse or use condoms for 2 days as she resumes her POP and it has time to take effect.

New Options on the Horizon

A new progestin-only pill (LF-111, 4mg drosperinone only; Leon Farma) finished its phase 3 clinical trial in August 2018 and has demonstrated higher efficacy in inhibiting ovulation as well as a longer window between doses, allowing for more flexibility in the timing of pills.[35,36]

Non-Contraceptive Benefits of CHC

Combined hormonal contraceptives have many non-contraceptive benefits and uses. They include regulation of the menstrual cycle or skipping the withdrawal bleed with continuous or semi-continuous use, decreasing overall menstrual blood loss, improving androgenic symptoms such as acne, and prevention of ovarian cancer. Studies have demonstrated that approximately 14% of women use contraception for non-contraceptive reasons only, with likely many more appreciating the added benefits.[37]

Additional benefits include reducing the risk of anemia, ovarian cancer, endometrial cancer, colorectal cancer, lymphatic and hematopoietic cancer, dysmenorrhea, menorrhagia, pelvic inflammatory disease, and benign breast disease.[33] The protective effects against endometrial, ovarian, and colorectal cancer continue for at least 30 years after discontinuation.[38] Research has shown that 31% of women use CHC for dysmenorrhea (cramps or pain), 28% for menstrual regulation or continuous use, 14% for acne, and 4% for endometriosis.[37] Physicians also prescribe CHC for treating hirsutism, menstrual migraine, and depression. Table 5 lists medical conditions improved by using CHC continuously, ie, without having a withdrawal bleed each month.[33]

Risks of CHC (the Ring, Patch, CHC pills)

Use of CHCs has risks, including VTE (which includes deep venous thrombosis), pulmonary embolism, stroke, breast cancer, cervical cancer, and elevated blood pressure. The CDC US MEC is a list of recommendations for using specific contraceptive methods based on specific medical conditions and medications. The CDC US MEC category 3 and 4 conditions are summarized in Table 6. The conditions can generally be divided into 3 categories: (1) conditions that place women at higher risk for VTE; (2) conditions in which subtle changes in liver enzymes could have harmful effects; and (3) medications that interfere with contraceptive efficacy or vice versa.

VTE

The contraindications to estrogen-containing contraception is mainly because of the risk for VTE, which is proportional to the estrogen dosage. Research has also shown that the risk for VTE differs by progestin with drosperinone, desogestrel and norgestimate associated with a greater risk than levonorgestrel. The risk for VTE in the general population is 1-2 in 10,000. On CHC pills the risk is 4-6 in 10,000 versus with pregnancy the risk is 8-10 in 10,000. The risk of VTE with any pill was lower than the risk of VTE with pregnancy.[39]

Cancer

Long-term use of oral contraceptives has been shown to decrease the risk for ovarian cancer, colon cancer, and endometrial cancer, but it has been shown to slightly increase the risk for breast cancer.[40] In large studies, ever-users had a 3% increase in relative risk of breast cancer compared to those who had never used CHCs, and women who were current users had a 24% increased risk with no increase with duration of use. However, this risk disappears 5 years after stopping CHCs.[40] A 2010 analysis of the Nurses Health Study of 116,000 female nurses aged 24 to 43 years found an increased risk of breast cancer only for those taking triphasic contraceptive pills.[41] Also, the risk might be an association confounded by delayed childbearing, as this also increases breast cancer risk. Newer data from a large homogeneous northern European population demonstrated a small overall increase in breast cancer risk, with 1 additional case of invasive breast cancer for every 7690 women using hormonal contraception.[42] Although the overall risk is low, it is unclear how to interpret this study because the study population is not generalizable to the United States, and investigators did not account for important confounders including alcohol consumption. Iversen et al[40] studied 46,022 women taking oral contraceptives for up to 44 years and concluded that "Most women who choose to use oral contraceptives do not expose themselves to long-term cancer harms; instead, with some cancers, many women benefit from important reductions of risk that persist for many years after stopping" and "the overall balance of cancer risk among past users of oral contraceptives was neutral with the increased risks counterbalanced by the endometrial, ovarian, and colorectal cancer benefits that persist at least 30 years." The rate of

Table 6
Condition categories 3/4 from CDC U.S. Medical Eligibility Criteria for combined hormonal contraceptives

Category 3: Condition for which theoretical or proven risks outweigh the advantages of using the method
Adequately controlled hypertension
Elevated blood pressure levels 140-159/90-99
Have deep vein thrombosis or pulmonary embolism, now or in the past
Multiple sclerosis *with* prolonged immobility
History of breast cancer without current disease for >5 years
Inflammatory bowel disease *with* increased risk of venous thromboembolism (eg, those with active or extensive disease, surgery, immobilization, corticosteroid use, vitamin deficiencies, fluid depletion)
Gallbladder disease only if treated medically
History of cholestasis related to combined oral contraception use
Acute viral hepatitis (initiation only)
Medications: some antiviral medications (fosamprenavir, ombitasvir, paritaprevir, ritonavir), certain anticonvulsants (phenytoin, carbamazepine, barbiturates, topiramate, oxcarbazepine), lamotrigine, antibiotics (rifampin)
Smoker (<15 cigarettes per day) *and* ≥35 years old
Category 4: Condition that represents an unacceptable health risk if contraceptive method is used
Elevated blood pressure levels ≥160/≥100
Vascular disease
History of DVT/PE *with* higher risk for recurrent DVT/PE (≥1 risk factor)
Major surgery *with* prolonged mobilization (without prolonged mobilization is category 2)
Known thrombogenic mutations (eg, factor V Leiden)
Current or history of ischemic heart disease
History of stroke
Complicated valvular heart disease *with* risk factors (hypertension, fibrillation)
Peripartum cardiomyopathy if <6 months ago
New York Heart Association functional class III or IV
Systemic lupus erythematosus *with* positive (or unknown) antiphospholipid antibodies
Migraine *with* aura
Current breast cancer
Diabetes with nephropathy, retinopathy, neuropathy, or other vascular disease of diabetes >20 years' duration
Hepatocellular adenoma
Malignant liver tumor
Severe (decompensated) cirrhosis
Complicated solid organ transplantation (graft failure, rejection, vasculopathy)
Smoker (≥15 cigarettes per day) *and* ≥35 years old

DVT, deep venous thrombosis; PE, pulmonary embolism.
Data from CDC US MEC for combined hormonal contraception. https://www.cdc.gov/reproductivehealth/contraception/mmwr/mec/appendixd.html. Accessed December 13, 2018.

invasive cervical cancer has been found to be 3.9 cases per 100,000 woman-years or 25% increased rate in women taking CHC pills compared to those not taking CHC.[40] However, this was before the advent of the human papillomavirus vaccine and may be confounded as women using contraceptive pills are more likely to be sexually active than women not using CHC pills.

Blood Pressure Elevation

Elevations in blood pressure often occur in women who initiate CHC. For women with normal blood pressure, initiating CHC typically does not cause development of true hypertension. In a small nonrandomized clinical trial, normotensive women who began taking an oral contraceptive containing 30 mcg EE and 150 mcg progestin had ambulatory blood pressure increased by approximately 8 mm Hg systolic and 6 mm Hg diastolic compared with no such increase in women beginning use of a copper IUD.[43] Combined hormonal contraceptives are CDC US MEC category 3 for women with well-controlled hypertension, and CHCs are CDC US MEC category 4 for women with poorly controlled hypertension. Elevated blood pressure as a result of taking CHCs is reversible upon stopping the CHCs. In a study of 1189 women, contraceptive pills containing norethindrone or desogestrel had little effect on blood pressure, but LNG did elevate blood pressure.[44]

Summary of Disadvantages to Specific Methods

The pill requires daily dosing, which is inconvenient and increases the likelihood of poor adherence. The patch has weekly dosing, has higher estrogen exposure with potential for greater VTE and other clotting risks, and can only be used for 12 weeks in a row versus continuous cycling for more than 12 weeks. The ring has monthly dosing versus longer dosing in LARC and increased vaginal discharge.

MANAGING COMMON PROBLEMS

Adverse Effects

Adverse effects are typically attributed to the estrogen, the progestational, or the androgenic effect of the progestin. Knowing the likely cause of the adverse effect (most commonly nausea and breakthrough bleeding) allows the practitioner to adjust the contraceptive pill or method appropriately. Table 7 reviews common adverse effects by hormonal source.

Table 7
Common side effects of combined oral contraception

Estrogenic	Progestin	Androgenic
Nausea and vomiting	Appetite	Depression
Breast tenderness	Breast tenderness	Fatigue
Bloating	Decreased libido	Increased libido
Telangiectasia	Changes in lipoproteins	Hirsutism
Thromboembolism	Changes in carbohydrate metabolism	Acne
Migraine vascular headache	Mood fluctuation	

Nausea

For women experiencing nausea related to CHC use, suggest that they take the pill with either with their largest meal of the day (usually dinner) or right before they go to bed (low incidence of waking up with nausea from medication). Should the nausea persist, prescribers can move the patient to a lower-dose estrogen formulation, but one that has at least 30 mcg EE for optimal bone health.[29]

Breakthrough Bleeding

Breakthrough bleeding (BTB) can occur in 7% to 10% of women using CHC, depending on which method and how long they have been on the method.[27] In a study of 6,724 women, BTB accounted for 13% of those who discontinued the CHC pill.[45] After ensuring that the patient is taking the medication at approximately the same time each day and that she is not taking magnesium or aluminum antacids (which interfere with absorption), first-line medication treatment of BTB is 600 mg ibuprofen up to 3 times per day with food (to avoid stomach upset) for up to 5 days. Failing ibuprofen, treatment consists of stronger progestin potency or lower estrogen (weighing risk of lower bone density versus side effects of BTB and adherence). Also keep in mind that sexually transmitted infections can cause spotting which patients might confuse for BTB.

Other Adverse Effects

For new or worsening headaches, which are related to the level of estrogen in the contraception method, consider changing to a method with a lower estrogen level. If the patient is using a drosperinone-based method, which has potential diuretic effects, and dehydration precipitates headaches, consider changing to a different progestin. Breast tenderness is common with CHC pills. Decreasing the level of estrogen or the progestational potency of the progestin (see Table 4 which shows progestin activity of common CHC pills) should alleviate breast tenderness. Vaginal dryness is associated with low estrogen, so increasing the estrogen may provide relief. Women taking CHCs can experience decreased libido, which is related to androgen strength, so changing the method to one containing a more androgenic progestin might help.

Nonadherence

Women report many reasons for not taking their birth control pills. Beyond common adverse effects such as nausea, the top 3 reasons women do not take their birth control pills are (1) they were away from home (12.9%); (2) they forgot (12.9%); and (3) they had no new pack (10.5%).[46] As physicians, we can mitigate these issues by offering an emergency pack (eg, for travel or if the patient forgets to refill at the pharmacy), being accessible to call in last-minute birth control prescriptions, encouraging the patient to download a medication reminder application to their smartphone, and writing a prescription for a

1 year's supply of contraceptives. Currently, 19 states require insurance to provide a year's supply of birth control at a time if written as such, although some require an initial 2- or 3-month supply before going to the entire year.[47]

SPECIAL CONSIDERATIONS

Oral Contraceptive Pills and Drug Interactions

Vitamin C increases estrogen. The OCPs decrease clearance of benzodiazepines, theophylline, aminophylline, corticosteroids, and tricyclic antidepressants, so you may want to decrease the dose of these medications because they will linger longer with OCPs. The OCPs increase the clearance of acetaminophen and aspirin, so you may need to increase your dosages of these medications. Medications that decrease OCP efficacy include anticonvulsants (specifically, phenytoin, phenobarbital, carbamazepine, oxcarbazepine, felbamate, ethosuximide, topiramate, primidone, vigabatrin) and antifungals (specifically, griseofulvin and itraconazole). Rifampin is the only antibiotic proven to decrease effectiveness of OCPs. Magnesium and aluminum antacids block the absorption of progestins.

Suicide and Hormonal Contraception

In 2017, Skovlund et al[48] published their findings following approximately 500,000 women for an average of 8.3 years, during which 6,999 first suicide attempts and 71 suicides were identified. Relative risk estimates for suicide attempts were 1.91 for CHC pills, 2.29 for POPs, 2.58 for vaginal ring, and 3.28 for the patch. The association between hormonal contraceptive use and a first suicide attempt peaked after 2 months of use. Adolescent women experienced the highest relative risk. However, the number needed to harm for suicide attempt is 1.4 per 1000 person-years and for suicide is 12 per 1,000,000 person-years.

Obesity and Hormonal Contraception

As obesity rates are climbing in all age groups, including adolescents, it is becoming more critical to evaluate contraception efficacy and safety within this population of women. Currently 21% of adolescent girls in the United States are obese, with the highest rates among non-Hispanic black teens, followed by Hispanic teens, among whom rates are increasing every year.[49] Data on contraceptive use demonstrate that obese women are more likely to not be using any type of contraception (adjusted odds ratio [OR] 1.53, 1.04-2.29) and more likely to experience unintended pregnancy (adjusted OR 1.67, 1.02-2.75).[50] Unintended pregnancy and delivery are higher risk in obese women, with studies demonstrating increased risk of birth defects, diabetes, hypertension, early delivery, and cesarean delivery, which must be considered in all contraceptive management.[51]

Sparse data exist on the effect of obesity on contraception efficacy and safety because earlier contraceptive trials excluded women with larger BMIs.[52] However, recent data have demonstrated decreased efficacy and increased risks for obese women, something that physicians may want to consider in their counseling of these women. Risk of pregnancy for women using CHC is up to 60% higher in women with BMI greater than 27 and 70% higher in women with BMI greater than 32.[53] For women using CHC pills, an FDA meta-analysis in 2015 of 7 studies had an overall adjusted hazard ratio of 1.44 or a 44% increased risk of unintended pregnancy in obese women compared with women of healthy weight. There also may be increased risks of complications, including VTE and metabolic syndrome, in obese women.

Because obese women were excluded from previous contraceptive patch and ring trials, there are sparse data regarding safety and efficacy alterations for these methods. Newer studies, including the study of the newer vaginal rings, include obesity without demonstrating a decrease in efficacy or safety in obese women. However, data are limited and data specific to obesity have not been specifically reported.[20]

AREAS FOR FUTURE RESEARCH

In summary, the contraceptive ring, patch, and pill are popular and effective options for preventing unplanned pregnancies and treating dysmenorrhea, anemia, and more. Several different options for and dosages of progestins and estrogen allow tailoring of oral CHC pills to a patient's individual response.

There is great potential for improvement in policy surrounding women's access to contraception. Research shows that with any copayments, women had a 9% increased risk of nonadherence.[54] Under the Affordable Care Act (ACA), all FDA-approved methods of contraception should be available with no copayments and no deductibles. Future research may study how this will change contraceptive method choice (such as long-activing reversible contraceptives) and long-term use among adolescents.

Funding for research on technological advances such as pill, patch, and ring reminder applications and gadgets that monitor pill adherence is needed. Per the American College of Obstetricians and Gynecologists policy statement that CHC should be over-the-counter, many companies have emerged to provide birth control by telemedicine.[55,56] How does online access to prescription contraception affect use, pregnancy rates, and sexually transmitted infection rates? More research on obesity and variation in response to various progestins by race/ethnicity is needed.

QUESTIONS

1. An 18-year-old female is heading off to college. She has no past medical history and does not smoke. Last week, she started taking a 35 mcg ethinyl estradiol and 0.25 mg norgestimate monophasic pill. She is having nausea with the pill. What is your next step in evaluating/addressing this adverse effect?
   A. Change her to a lower-dose estrogen pill.
   B. Change her to a higher-dose estrogen pill.
   C. Ask her when she is taking her pill and whether she taking it with food.
   D. Try a method without estrogen.
   E. Change her to a different progestin.
2. After 2 months of taking this oral contraceptive pill (OCP), she is having breakthrough bleeding. After making sure that she is taking it at the same time every day and that she is not taking a medication that would affect absorption, what should you do next to manage this situation?
   A. Reassure her that this is normal and things will get better.
   B. Suggest a trial of ibuprofen 600 mg TID with food for up to 5 days.
   C. Change her to a progestin with a greater progestational effect.
   D. Decrease the estrogen in the OCP.
3. Which one of the following progestins has the least androgenic effect?
   A. Levonorgestrel
   B. Norgestimate
   C. Drosperinone
4. Which one of the following progestins has the most androgenic effect?
   A. Levonorgestrel
   B. Norgestimate
   C. Drosperinone
5. An adolescent woman asks to be put on low-dose birth control pills. As her physician who carefully read this article, you suggest that she have at least 30 mcg ethinyl estradiol in her birth control pill. Why?
   A. Less than 30 mcg ethinyl estradiol results in more nausea for women of childbearing age.
   B. Less than 30 mcg ethinyl estradiol is associated with greater risk for blood clots in adolescents.
   C. Less than 30 mcg ethinyl estradiol results in lower bone density for women of bone density accrual age.

(See pages 200-201 for answers.)

References

1. Abma JC, Martinez GM. Sexual activity and contraceptive use among teenagers in the United States, 2011-2015. *Natl Health Stat Report*. 2017;104:1-23
2. Finer LB, Zolna MR. Declines in unintended pregnancy in the United States, 2008-2011. *N Engl J Med*. 2016;374:843-852
3. Martin JA, Hamilton BE, Osterman MJK, Driscoll AK, Drake P. Births: final data for 2016. *Natl Vital Stat Rep*. 2018;67:1-55
4. Sedgh G, Finer LB, Bankole A, Eilers MA, Singh S. Adolescent pregnancy, birth, and abortion rates across countries: levels and recent trends. *J Adolesc Health*. 2015;56:223-230
5. Mestad R, Secura G, Allsworth JE, Madden T, Zhao Q, Peipert JF. Acceptance of long-acting reversible contraceptive methods by adolescent participants in the Contraceptive CHOICE Project. *Contraception*. 2011;84:493-498
6. Curtis KM, Jatlaoui TC, Tepper NK, et al. U.S. Selected Practice Recommendations for Contraceptive Use, 2016. *MMWR Recomm Rep*. 2016;65(No. RR-4):1–66
7. Peipert JF, Madden T, Allsworth JE, Secura GM. Preventing unintended pregnancies by providing no-cost contraception. *Obstet Gynecol*. 2012;120:1291-1297
8. Dehlendorf C, Ruskin R, Grumbach K, et al. Recommendations for intrauterine contraception: a randomized trial of the effects of patients' race/ethnicity and socioeconomic status. *Am J Obstet Gynecol*. 2010;203:319.e1-e8
9. Ott MA, Sucato GS; American Academy of Pediatrics Committee on Adolescence. Contraception for adolescents. *Pediatrics*. 2014;134:e1257-e1281
10. Tepper NK, Krashin JW, Curtis KM, Cox S, Whiteman MK. Update to CDC's U.S. Medical Eligibility Criteria for Contraceptive Use, 2016: revised recommendations for the use of hormonal contraception among women at high risk for HIV infection. *MMWR Morb Mortal Wkly Rep*. 2017;66:990-994
11. Edelman A, Micks E, Gallo MF, Jensen JT, Grimes DA. Continuous or extended cycle vs. cyclic use of combined hormonal contraceptives for contraception. *Cochrane Database Syst Rev*. 2014;7:CD004695
12. NuvaRing [package insert]. Whitehouse Station, NJ: Merck & Co., Inc; 2005
13. Bitzer J. The vaginal ring (NuvaRing) for contraception in adolescent women. *Gynecol Endocrinol*. 2012;28:125-129
14. Veres S, Miller L, Burington B. A comparison between the vaginal ring and oral contraceptives. *Obstet Gynecol*. 2004;104:555-563
15. Mohamed AM, El-Sherbiny WS, Mostafa WA. Combined contraceptive ring versus combined oral contraceptive (30-mug ethinylestradiol and 3-mg drospirenone). *Int J Gynaecol Obstet*. 2011;114(2):145-148.
16. Tuppurainen M, Klimscheffskij R, Venhola M, Dieben TO. The combined contraceptive vaginal ring (NuvaRing) and lipid metabolism: a comparative study. *Contraception*. 2004;69(5):389-394
17. Verhoeven CH, Dieben TO. The combined contraceptive vaginal ring, NuvaRing, and tampon co-usage. *Contraception*. 2004;69:197-199
18. Verhoeven CH, van den Heuvel MW, Mulders TM, Dieben TO. The contraceptive vaginal ring, NuvaRing, and antimycotic co-medication. *Contraception*. 2004;69:129-132
19. Population Council. FDA approves the first one-year contraceptive fully under a woman's control. https://www.popcouncil.org/news/fda-approves-the-first-one-year-contraceptive-fully-under-a-womans-control. Published August 10, 2018. Accessed November 15, 2018
20. Annovera [package insert]. New York, NY: Population Council; 2018
21. Jensen JT, Edelman AB, Chen BA, et al. Continuous dosing of a novel contraceptive vaginal ring releasing Nestorone and estradiol: pharmacokinetics from a dose-finding study. *Contraception*. 2018;97:422-427

22. Lavelanet AF, Rybin D, White KO. The pharmacokinetics of 12-week continuous contraceptive patch use. *Contraception*. 2017;95:578-585
23. Hatcher RA, Nelson AI, Trussell J, et al, eds. *Contraceptive Technology*. 21st ed. New York, NY: Ayer Company Publishers, Inc; 2018
24. Zieman M, Guillebaud J, Weisberg E, et al. Contraceptive efficacy and cycle control with the Ortho Evra/Evra transdermal system: the analysis of pooled data. *Fertil Steril*. 2002;77(2 Suppl 2):S13-18
25. Xulane [package insert]. Morgantown, WV: Mylan Pharmaceuticals Inc; 2001
26. Rubinstein ML, Halpern-Felsher BL, Irwin CE Jr. An evaluation of the use of the transdermal contraceptive patch in adolescents. *J Adolesc Health*. 2004;34:395-401
27. Audet MC, Moreau M, Koltun WD, et al. Evaluation of contraceptive efficacy and cycle control of a transdermal contraceptive patch vs an oral contraceptive: a randomized controlled trial. *JAMA*. 2001;285(18):2347-2354
28. Smallwood GH, Meador ML, Lenihan JP, et al. Efficacy and safety of a transdermal contraceptive system. *Obstet Gynecol*. 2001;98(5 Pt 1):799-805
29. Scholes D, Ichikawa L, LaCroix AZ, et al. Oral contraceptive use and bone density in adolescent and young adult women. *Contraception*. 2010;81:35-40
30. Glasier AF, Smith KB, van der Spuy ZM, et al. Amenorrhea associated with contraception-an international study on acceptability. *Contraception*. 2003;67:1-8
31. Gladwell M. Annals of Medicine, "John Rock's Error". *The New Yorker*. Vol March 13, 2000.
32. Countinho EM SS. *Is Menstruation Obsolete?* New York, NY: Oxford University Press; 1999
33. Altshuler AL, Hillard PJ. Menstrual suppression for adolescents. *Curr Opin Obstet Gynecol*. 2014;26(5):323-331
34. American College of Obsetricians and Gynecologists. Progestin-Only Hormonal Birth Control: Pill and Injection. March 2018; https://www.acog.org/Patients/FAQs/Progestin-Only-Hormonal-Birth-Control-Pill-and-Injection?IsMobileSet=false–work. Accessed November 18, 2018
35. Archer DF, Ahrendt HJ, Drouin D. Drospirenone-only oral contraceptive: results from a multi-center noncomparative trial of efficacy, safety and tolerability. *Contraception*. 2015;92:439-444
36. Duijkers IJM, Heger-Mahn D, Drouin D, Colli E, Skouby S. Maintenance of ovulation inhibition with a new progestogen-only pill containing drospirenone after scheduled 24-h delays in pill intake. *Contraception*. 2016;93:303-309
37. Jones RK. *Beyond Birth Control: The Overlooked Benefits of Oral Contraceptive Pills*. New York: Guttmacher Institute; 2011. https://www.guttmacher.org/report/beyond-birth-control-overlooked-benefits-oral-contraceptive-pills. Published November 2011. Accessed November 15, 2018
38. Gierisch JM, Coeytaux RR, Urrutia RP, et al. Oral contraceptive use and risk of breast, cervical, colorectal, and endometrial cancers: a systematic review. *Cancer Epidemiol Biomarkers Prev*. 2013;22(11):1931-1943
39. van Hylckama Vlieg A, Helmerhorst FM, Vandenbroucke JP, Doggen CJ, Rosendaal FR. The venous thrombotic risk of oral contraceptives, effects of oestrogen dose and progestogen type: results of the MEGA case-control study. *BMJ*. 2009;339:b2921
40. Iversen L, Sivasubramaniam S, Lee AJ, Fielding S, Hannaford PC. Lifetime cancer risk and combined oral contraceptives: the Royal College of General Practitioners' Oral Contraception Study. *Am J Obstet Gynecol*. 2017;216:580.e1-580.e9
41. Beaber EF, Buist DS, Barlow WE, Malone KE, Reed SD, Li CI. Recent oral contraceptive use by formulation and breast cancer risk among women 20 to 49 years of age. *Cancer Res*. 2014;74(15):4078-4089
42. Morch LS, Skovlund CW, Hannaford PC, et al. Contemporary hormonal contraception and the risk of breast cancer. *N Engl J Med*. 2017;377:2228-2239
43. Cardoso F, Polonia J, Santos A, Silva-Carvalho J, Ferreira-de-Almeida J. Low-dose oral contraceptives and 24-hour ambulatory blood pressure. *Int J Gynaecol Obstet*. 1997;59:237-243
44. Godsland IF, Walton C, Felton C, Proudler A, Patel A, Wynn V. Insulin resistance, secretion, and metabolism in users of oral contraceptives. *J Clin Endocrinol Metab*. 1992;74:64-70
45. Moreau C, Cleland K, Trussell J. Contraceptive discontinuation attributed to method dissatisfaction in the United States. *Contraception*. 2007;76(4):267-272

46. Smith JD, Oakley D. Why do women miss oral contraceptive pills? An analysis of women's self-described reasons for missed pills. *J Midwifery Womens Health*. 2005;50:380-385
47. At a glance: coverage for an extended supply of contraception. Power To Decide. August 2018. https://powertodecide.org/system/files/resources/primary-download/extended-supply-contraception.pdf. Accessed November 15, 2018
48. Skovlund CW, Morch LS, Kessing LV, Lange T, Lidegaard O. Association of hormonal contraception with suicide attempts and suicides. *Am J Psychiatry*. 2018;175:336-342
49. Hales CM, Carroll MD, Fryar CD, Ogden CL. Prevalence of obesity among adults and youth, 2015-2016. *NCHS Data Brief*. 2017;288:1-8
50. Nguyen BT, Elia JL, Ha CY, Kaneshiro BE. Pregnancy intention and contraceptive use among women by class of obesity: results from the 2006-2010 and 2011-2013 National Survey of Family Growth. *Womens Health Issues*. 2018;28:51-58
51. ACOG Practice Bulletin No. 156: obesity in pregnancy. *Obstet Gynecol*. 2015;126:e112-e126
52. Edelman A, Trussell J, Aiken ARA, et al. The emerging role of obesity in short-acting hormonal contraceptive effectiveness. *Contraception*. 2018;97:371-377
53. Holt VL, Cushing-Haugen KL, Daling JR. Body weight and risk of oral contraceptive failure. *Obstet Gynecol*. 2002;99:820-827
54. Marshall C, Schmittdiel J, Chandra M, Calhoun A, Raine-Bennett T. The relationship between prescription copayments and contraceptive adherence in a new-user cohort. *Med Care*. 2018;56: 577-582
55. American College of Obstetricians and Gynecologists Committee on Gynecologic Practice. Committee Opinion No. 544: over-the-counter access to oral contraceptives. *Obstet Gynecol*. 2012;120:1527-1531
56. Dennis A, Grossman D. Barriers to contraception and interest in over-the-counter access among low-income women: a qualitative study. *Perspect Sex Reprod Health*. 2012;44:84-91

Adolesc Med 030 (2019) 82–101

Depo-Provera: Is It Still a Good Option for Adolescents?

Andrea E. Bonny, MD[a*]; Hannah L.H. Lange, MPH[b]

[a]*Associate Professor of Pediatrics, The Ohio State University College of Medicine, Columbus, Ohio, Research Director, Division of Adolescent Medicine, Nationwide Children's Hospital, Columbus, Ohio;* [b]*Clinical Research Team Lead, Division of Adolescent Medicine, Nationwide Children's Hospital, Columbus, Ohio*

LEARNING OBJECTIVES

After reviewing this article, the reader should be able to:

1. Summarize the risks and benefits of DMPA as a contraceptive method for adolescents
2. Describe appropriate clinical management of DMPA-associated adverse effects in adolescents
3. Recognize the potential benefits of DMPA-SC 104 mg for the adolescent patient

INTRODUCTION

Since its introduction, the progestin-only injectable steroid Depo-Provera, or depot medroxyprogesterone acetate (DMPA), has weathered controversy.[1] Despite this, it has remained a popular contraceptive method among adolescents and has contributed to declining teen pregnancy rates.[2-4] Between 2011 and 2015, 17.2% of sexually experienced female teenagers had ever used Depo-Provera, approximately double the rate of use in 1995.[2,3] High efficacy, ease of use, and potential for anonymity are several attributes that make DMPA appealing for adolescents.[5] As an injectable method, DMPA provides "intermediate-acting" reversible contraception while avoiding the need for daily/weekly dosing

*Corresponding author
E-mail address: andrea.bonny@nationwidechildrens.org

 ISSN 1934-4287

or device insertion. It fills an important contraceptive niche as some adolescents are uncomfortable with contraceptive methods requiring placement of a foreign body.[6-8]

CONTROVERSIAL HISTORY

DMPA was initially synthesized in 1954 (Figure 1) and received United States (US) Food and Drug Administration (FDA) approval in 1969 for the treatment of uterine and kidney cancers. By the early 1960s, it was evident that DMPA provided effective contraception, and it was used off-label by many thousands of women in the United States for this purpose. By 1980, more than 80 developed and developing countries had approved DMPA as a contraceptive agent, but approval was delayed in the United States and United Kingdom. In 1974 and 1978, the Obstetrics & Gynecology and the Biometric & Epidemiology Methodology Committees of the US FDA recommended registration of DMPA as a contraceptive. Both times, the FDA Commissioner rejected the registration because of concerns about cancer in animals dosed with high levels of DMPA. During this time, DMPA continued to be available in the United States for cancer-related therapeutic uses.

The unwillingness of the FDA to widen DMPA's application served as a lightning rod for both popular and scientific controversy.[1] Some acclaimed DMPA as a much wanted "long-acting" contraceptive that would protect women, increase contraceptive choices, and assist individuals and societies with fertility goals. Others rejected it as an example of foisting unsolicited and questionable therapies, particularly among populations of developing countries, with no concern for individual health. Ultimately on October 29, 1992, the FDA approved Depo-Provera as an intramuscular contraceptive agent. By then, it had been used by more than 30 million women worldwide for this purpose.

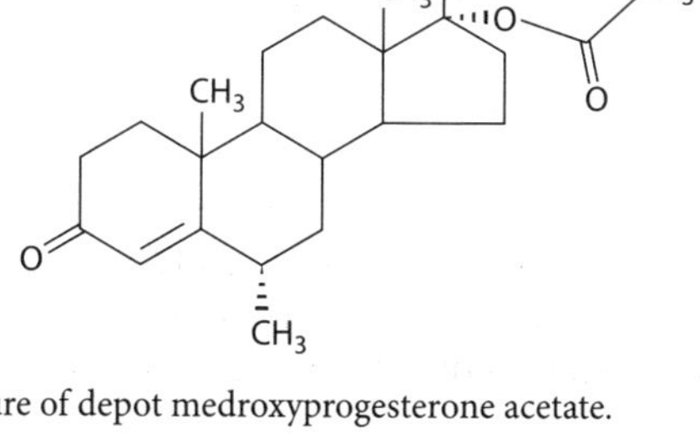

Fig 1. Molecular structure of depot medroxyprogesterone acetate.

ESTABLISHMENT OF DMPA DOSE

Despite early evidence that lower doses could provide effective contraception, the contraceptive dose of DMPA was initially established as 150 mg given intramuscularly (IM) every 12 weeks.[9-11] Early studies of DMPA-IM 150 mg consistently found that this dose inhibited formation of a functional corpus luteum for a prolonged (>200 days) period of time.[10] Among Mexican women, DMPA IM doses as low as 25 mg were found to provide effective contraception for at least 3 months.[9] Among Thai women, although DMPA-IM 100 mg was found to be effective for at least 90 days, doses of 25 and 50 mg were not.[11] In a multicenter, phase III, comparative clinical trial of DMPA sponsored by the World Health Organization, little difference in efficacy and safety was found between DMPA-IM 150 mg and 100 mg. However, 2 pregnancies occurred in women receiving 100 mg IM (Pearl index = 0.44 per 100 woman-years), whereas none occurred in those who received 150 mg.[12] This difference likely contributed to the ultimate recommendation of a 3-monthly dose of DMPA-IM 150 mg.

In 2004, a lower-dose subcutaneous (SC) formulation of DMPA was released (Depo-subQ Provera 104 [DMPA-SC]).[13] Goals of the lower-dose DMPA-SC were to maintain contraceptive efficacy while minimizing adverse effects and hastening return to cyclic ovulation through dose reduction. However, delayed return to fertility is still observed with DMPA-SC.[14] Median time for return to ovulation with DMPA-SC is 30 weeks, with a cumulative rate of return to ovulation of 97.4% at 12 months.[14] In comparison, median time to conception with DMPA-IM 150 mg is 10 months (range 4-31 months).[15] Although data are still emerging, adverse effect profiles seem similar between the 2 formulations.[16]

In comparison to DMPA-IM, DMPA-SC has the added benefit of potential for self-administration at home. Recent evidence finds that many adolescents are interested in and capable of DMPA-SC self-administration.[17,18] Although self-injection may not be appropriate for all adolescents who utilize DMPA, the potential for discreet use and user control inherent in the practice of self-injection aligns with adolescent priorities for contraceptive services.[18] Emerging data find that self-administration of DMPA-SC can improve contraceptive continuation, even among adolescents, and investigators have called for wider availability of the DMPA-SC self-administration option.[19]

POTENTIAL ADVERSE EFFECTS

Adverse effects continue to be a major reason for discontinuation of DMPA use. Unwanted weight gain, irregular uterine bleeding, and bone mineral density (BMD) loss are especially pertinent to adolescents. However, with appropriate patient screening and management, adverse effects can be kept to a minimum.

BONE MINERAL DENSITY LOSS

Adolescence and young adulthood represent a critical time for bone accumulation.[20] In girls, peak bone mineral accrual occurs at 12.5 ± 0.9 years, and 26% of adult BMD is accumulated at this time.[21-23] From 80% to 90% of bone mineral content is achieved by 16 years of age, and 99% of peak bone mineral content is reached by 26 years.[24-28] Sex steroids, particularly estrogen, are critical players in bone development. Estradiol inhibits osteoclasts, exerting an antiresorptive effect on bone.[29] As a progestin-only contraceptive, DMPA creates a low estrogen environment, which can have a negative effect on bone health.[30]

Although cross-sectional studies found no significant differences in BMD between adolescent females using DMPA compared to those using no hormonal method or combined oral contraceptives (COCs),[31,32] longitudinal studies have consistently noted BMD losses in the hip and spine among adolescent females using DMPA.[33-37] Busen et al[33] noted a mean loss of BMD of -3.31% ($P = .01$) at the femoral neck and -3.52% ($P = .02$) at the lumbar spine among 6 adolescents, aged 15 to 19 years, at 1 year of DMPA use. Lara-Torre et al[35] conducted a prospective study of 77 adolescent females aged 12 to 21 years using DMPA or no hormonal contraceptive method. Lumbar spine BMD measurements were obtained at 6-month intervals for 24 months. Adolescents using DMPA experienced a loss in lumbar spine BMD over the course of the study (mean loss -1.6% at 1 year and -1.8% at 2 years). In contrast, those using no hormonal contraception experienced increases in lumbar spine BMD over the same time period (mean gain 2.4% at 1 year and 5.9% at 2 years). At all follow-up time points, significant differences in lumbar spine BMD were evident between adolescents using DMPA compared to those using no hormonal contraception.[35]

Cromer et al[34,36,37] conducted 2 prospective studies of adolescents using DMPA. In an earlier study that prospectively followed 32 female adolescents aged 12 to 21 years using DMPA or no hormonal contraceptive method, significant group differences in lumbar spine BMD changes were found at 1 and 2 years. Adolescents using DMPA saw mean lumbar spine BMD changes of -1.5% at 1 year and -3.1% at 2 years; those using no hormonal contraception saw mean lumbar spine BMD increases of 2.9% and 9.5% at 1 and 2 years.[34] In a larger study of 370 adolescent females aged 12 to 18 years, Cromer at al[36] again found decreases in BMD in those using DMPA with concomitant increases in BMD in the control group using no hormonal contraception. At 1 year, adolescents using DMPA had a mean BMD change of -1.4% at the lumbar spine and -2.2% at the femoral neck, whereas those in the control group saw increases of 3.8% at the lumbar spine and 2.3% at the femoral neck.[36] At 2 years, adolescents using DMPA had a mean BMD change of -1.5% at the lumbar spine and -5.2% at the femoral neck, whereas those in the control group saw increases of 6.3% at the lumbar spine and 3.8% at the femoral neck. However, Cromer et al[37] noted that the clinical significance of the BMD loss seen at 2 years among those using DMPA was "mitigated by slowed loss after the first year…and general maintenance of bone density values within the normal range."

Of interest, Beksinska et al[38] found no difference in BMD increases among adolescent females aged 15 to 19 years using DMPA compared to nonusers. However, this 5-year longitudinal study measured BMD at the distal radius rather than the hip or lumbar spine. Annum BMD increases were 1.39% in DMPA users and 1.49% in nonusers. Tharnprisarn and Taneepanichskul[32] suggested that different skeletal sites vary in their sensitivity to hormonally associated BMD changes.

Mitigating BMD Loss

As described in the section on Bone Mineral Density Loss, the mechanism of DMPA-associated bone loss has generally been thought to be estrogen deficiency caused by hypothalamic-pituitary-ovarian axis suppression. Two randomized controlled trials found that supplementation with estrogen mitigates bone losses in adult[39] and adolescent[40] females using DMPA. However, factors other than low estrogen also seem to be at play. Body weight is generally a positive predictor of bone strength,[41] and body fat and lean mass during childhood and adolescence are positively correlated with BMD.[42,43] In adolescents, body weight continues to be highly correlated with both spine and femoral neck BMD regardless of DMPA use.[44] Harel et al[45] found that adequate calcium intake (28 servings or more per week) was associated with significantly less BMD loss at both the femoral neck and total hip among adolescents using DMPA. Adequate calcium and vitamin D intake should be encouraged in adolescents using this contraceptive method. Current dietary guidelines recommend 1300 mg/day of calcium and 600 IU/day of vitamin D for all adolescent females aged 14 to 18 years.[46]

Newer evidence finds that DMPA dose may also affect BMD losses. In adult women, decreased losses in spine BMD were evident at 12 months among those receiving DMPA-SC 104 mg compared to those receiving DMPA-IM 150 mg (-2.4% DMPA-SC vs -3.4% DMPA-IM; P = .02); however, these differences did not persist after 2 and 3 years of DMPA use.[47] Lange et al[48] conducted a 48-week randomized trial of 3 doses of DMPA-IM (150, 104, and 75 mg) in 34 adolescent females aged 12 to 21 years.[48] At 48 weeks, no significant decreases in BMD at any measured site were evident among those receiving DMPA-IM 75 mg. Participants receiving DMPA-IM 104 mg experienced significant BMD loss only in the lumbar spine (-3.1%; P <.01), whereas those receiving DMPA-IM 150 mg had significant decreases in BMD at all measured anatomic sites (-4.0% lumbar spine, -3.0% femoral neck, -4.0% total hip; all P <.05).[48] This study provided the first evidence of a dose–response relationship between DMPA-IM dose and

BMD loss in adolescents. Whether this finding extends to DMPA-SC has not yet been studied. Of note, 45% of adolescents in this study who were receiving DMPA-IM 75 mg required dose escalation to maintain contraceptive efficacy, whereas no participants receiving 104 or 150 mg required a dose change. The potential benefit of decreased DMPA dose must always be balanced with the risk of contraceptive efficacy loss.

Recovery of BMD Loss

In addition to mitigating BMD losses experienced while using DMPA, there is the crucial issue of recovery of BMD losses after discontinuation of the method. Data demonstrate that BMD loss in female adolescents is substantially or fully reversible in most girls 1 to 2 years after discontinuation of the method.[45,49,50] Two longitudinal studies found that after discontinuation of DMPA, mean BMD values increased more rapidly for DMPA users compared to nonusers.[49,50] After DMPA discontinuation, Scholes et al[49] reported annualized mean percentage change in BMD of 1.34% versus -0.19% at the hip, 2.86% versus 1.32% at the spine, and 3.56% versus 0.88% in whole body among DMPA users and nonusers, respectively. Similarly, after DMPA discontinuation, Shen et al[50] reported annualized mean percentage change in BMD of 1.72% versus 0.94% at the spine and 1.63% versus 0.91% at the femoral neck among DMPA users and nonusers.

Harel et al[45] found that within 60 weeks of discontinuation of DMPA, mean lumbar spine BMD returned to baseline levels, and that by 240 weeks after DMPA mean lumbar spine BMD was 4.7% above baseline value. Recovery was slower at the hip, with mean total hip and femoral neck BMD values recovering to baseline at 240 and 180 weeks after DMPA discontinuation, respectively.[45] Of note, BMD recovery was overall slower and less robust among participants with ≥5% BMD loss compared to those with less than 5% loss.[45] Factors associated with ≥5% BMD loss included lower body mass index (BMI) and calcium intake and greater alcohol use, reminding clinicians of the importance of discussing overall health (eg, dietary intake, substance use) with adolescent contraceptive users.[51]

Clinical Significance of BMD Findings in Adolescents

In 2004, the FDA issued a boxed warning for DMPA concerning BMD loss.[52] This warning stated that women who use DMPA may lose significant BMD, and that the loss increases with longer duration of use and may not be reversible. The warning further stated that it is unknown whether DMPA use in adolescence or early adulthood will reduce peak bone mass. The warning recommends that DMPA should not be used for more than 2 years unless other methods of contraception are deemed inadequate.[52]

However, a key concept to consider when interpreting the literature on DMPA and BMD loss is whether the risk of osteoporotic fragility fractures is increased by DMPA use. The predominant literature to date has examined BMD as a surrogate marker for future fragility fracture risk. Bone strength depends not only on BMD but also on other bone qualities (eg, bone geometry and architecture) that are not captured in common measurements of BMD.[45] Previous studies of adolescents have not been powered to assess fragility fractures as a clinical endpoint. In addition, age is an important predictor of fracture risk as well as bone mass, so small differences in BMD (eg, 5%-10%) that can affect the risk of fracture in postmenopausal women have minimal effect on fracture rate in women younger than 45 years.[53] Some experts have called for the removal of the FDA boxed warning for DMPA, citing both lack of convincing evidence that DMPA use is linked to fracture risk and clinical recommendations based on invalid surrogate endpoints.[54]

In 2006, the Society for Adolescent Health and Medicine published a position paper on the boxed warning for DMPA.[55] The statement stressed the need to balance the physical and socioeconomic costs of adolescent pregnancy with DMPA effect on bone. Clinical guidelines recommend that clinicians (1) continue to prescribe DMPA to adolescents with full discussion of risks and benefits; (2) inform patients of the potential risk for BMD loss; (3) understand each patient's individual risk profile for osteopenia while using DMPA; (4) consider BMD monitoring, particularly if conditions of concern (eg, low body weight) apply to a given patient; (5) not restrict duration of use to 2 years; (6) recommend adequate daily calcium and vitamin D intake and weight-bearing exercise to adolescents using DMPA; and (7) consider estrogen supplementation in adolescents with osteopenia who are doing well on DMPA and have no contraindications to estrogen. Overall, there is no indication for BMD monitoring in an otherwise healthy adolescent using DMPA. However, clinicians may consider BMD assessment before DMPA initiation in adolescents with other risk factors for low BMD.

In 2014, the American College of Obstetricians and Gynecologists issued a committee opinion reiterating that clinicians should not limit DMPA use to 2 years, as doing so could disproportionately affect adolescents who value the privacy and convenience of DMPA. In addition, the committee highlighted that the health and social consequences of unintended pregnancy are particularly high in adolescence.[56] Per the U.S. Medical Eligibility Criteria for Contraceptive Use, adolescence (from menarche to $<$18 years) is a category 2 condition in which the advantages of DMPA use generally outweigh the risks in this age group.[57]

WEIGHT CHANGES

Weight gain is a prominent concern for adolescents considering DMPA use. This concern is reported in up to 54% of adolescents who use this method[58-62] and is cited as a major reason for method discontinuation.[63] Only 9% of adolescents who discontinue DMPA use because of weight concerns will restart this method compared to 80% who discontinue because of missed appointments.[64]

Despite this, weight gain has not been a universal finding in research studies of adolescents using this contraceptive. Reported mean weight gain at 1 year among adolescents using DMPA varies widely (range 0.05-4.44 kg).[65,66] Data are limited by small sample sizes, lack of longitudinal data, and inadequate control groups.[67] Additionally, the causal association between contraceptive use and weight is difficult to study, given that some weight gain is normal and appropriate during adolescence.

Excessive weight gain rather than mean weight gain may be a better paradigm for examining DMPA-associated weight gain. Risser et al[59] compared weight change at 1 year between adolescents who were using DMPA and those using COC. Although mean weight gain was not different between groups, a significantly higher percentage of those using DMPA gained more than 10% of baseline body weight (25% DMPA vs 7% COC; $P = .006$). More recent studies in both adults and adolescents have provided additional evidence that approximately 1 in 4 females are at risk for excessive DMPA-associated weight gain.[61,62]

Risk Factors for Weight Gain

Baseline obesity status has been reported as a potential risk factor for excessive weight gain among adolescents using DMPA.[59,60,68] In contrast, no association between baseline weight and DMPA-associated weight gain has been generally seen in adult women.[69] Two retrospective studies in adolescents found that overweight at time of DMPA initiation was associated with greater weight gain.[59,60] Bonny et al[68] duplicated this finding in a prospective study of adolescents initiating DMPA or no hormonal contraception. At 18 months, obese adolescents using DMPA had gained significantly more weight (9.5 kg) than their obese counterparts using no hormonal contraception (3.1 kg). In contrast, there was no difference in weight gain at this time point between non-obese females using DMPA (4.0 kg) or no hormonal contraception (3.5 kg). Despite this evidence in adolescents, obesity is still a U.S. Medical Eligibility Criteria for Contraceptive Use category 2 condition in this age group; that is, the advantages of DMPA use generally outweigh the risks.[57]

Racial and ethnic differences in DMPA-associated weight gain have also been observed in adolescents. In a prospective study, Polaneczky et al[64] found that black adolescents gained significantly more weight at 11.1 months of DMPA use (7.4 pounds) compared to Hispanic (2.3 pounds) and white (-2.9 pounds) females. Similarly, Bonny et al[70] identified racial differences in weight gain at 6 months of DMPA use (2.9 kg black vs 0.9 kg white adolescents). Hispanic ethnicity was found to confer protection against weight gain over 6 months in a sample of adolescents using DMPA.[71] It is important to note, however, that the strength of these findings is insufficient to preclude clinicians from recommending DMPA based on racial or ethnic background.

Unlike the observed dose-response relationship between DMPA dose and BMD (see section on Bone Mineral Density Loss), the dose of DMPA does not seem to affect weight gain, but data are limited. In an early study, Harel et al[72] found that early second injection of DMPA predisposed to more weight gain than receipt of the second DMPA injection at the standard 3-month interval, suggesting that higher exposure to DMPA may be associated with greater weight gain. In contrast, Templeman et al[66] found no significant difference in weight between adolescents receiving DMPA at 3-month intervals compared to those receiving monthly injections for 3 doses followed by 3-month dosing. A randomized clinical trial of 3 doses of DMPA found no differences in mean weight change or percentage of participants gaining more than 5% over baseline at 6 months between adolescents receiving 150, 104, or 75 mg IM at 12-week intervals.[48]

Pharmacokinetic profile may be more important than DMPA dose for predicting weight gain while using DMPA. An exploration of DMPA pharmacokinetics among 40 adolescents aged 12 to 21 years starting DMPA reported differing pharmacokinetic profiles for those with and those without a 10% annualized percentage increase in BMI.[73] Those with 10% or greater annualized increase in BMI had a lower maximum DMPA concentration and flatter medroxyprogesterone concentration time curve representing delayed DMPA clearance. An elimination rate constant less than 0.0221 ng/mL/day was the most significant predictor of an annualized BMI increase of 10% or more in this study.

Several studies have examined the relationship between early weight gain and future weight gain while using DMPA. Risser et al[59] noted that adolescents who gained more than 5% of baseline weight at 3 months of DMPA use were at high risk for gaining even more weight by 1 year. Le et al[61] explored the association between early weight gain, defined as more than 5% over baseline at 6 months, and future weight gain in adult females using DMPA. They found early weight gain was highly predictive of continued excessive weight gain. After adjusting for potential confounders, those with early weight gain went on to gain approximately 7.03 kg more over 36 months (95% confidence interval 5.519–8.541; $P < .001$) compared to women with 5% or less weight increase at 6 months. The findings of Le et al[61] were replicated in adolescents initiating DMPA.[62] Despite no significant difference in baseline BMI, adolescents with early weight gain had a significantly higher BMI at 18 months of DMPA use (32.1 kg/m^2 early weight gainers vs 25.7 kg/m^2 non-early weight gainers). To date, early weight gain continues to be the most robust and clinically useful predictor of weight gain profile while using DMPA. Patients who experience 5% or less weight gain at 6 months can likely be reassured regarding their future risk for weight gain. These patients should continue to receive routine diet and exercise counseling.

Although 6-month weight gain is helpful, a baseline biomarker of risk would be able to identify individuals before DMPA initiation. To this end, our investigative team explored biologic predictors of DMPA-associated weight gain in adolescents. In a small pilot study, we found that serum adiponectin concentration, independent of baseline adiposity, was a potentially useful biologic marker for risk of excessive weight gain.[71] Decreased serum adiponectin seemed to place adolescents at greater risk for DMPA-associated weight gain, which may be of particular concern for obese adolescents. However, more studies in larger and more diverse cohorts are needed before changes are made in clinical practice.

Body Composition Changes During DMPA Use

Weight gain during DMPA use is entirely caused by increases in total body fat. Several studies in adult women have documented significant increases in body fat among those using DMPA compared to those using COC or using a no hormonal contraceptive method.[69,74,75] A small longitudinal study of adolescents receiving hormonal contraception similarly found that DMPA use was associated with significant increases in total body fat with concomitant decreases in lean body mass.[76] At 6 months, adolescents receiving DMPA experienced a 10% increase in total body fat compared to a 1% increase among those on no hormonal contraception. Interestingly, this study found some evidence that supplemental estrogen via monthly estradiol injections mitigated DMPA-associated body composition changes. Whether body composition changes are reversible after DMPA cessation and their long-term clinical significance are not known.

Dietary Behaviors and Weight Gain During DMPA Use

Although DMPA-associated weight gain has been postulated to be related to increased appetite and subsequent increased caloric intake,[77] research has not supported this mechanism. A prospective, longitudinal study of adolescent females initiating DMPA found no association between appetite and weight changes. In fact, mean appetite scores decreased among study participants despite concomitant increases in weight, and drops in appetite scores were largest among those who experienced the most weight gain.[70] In a 1-year prospective observational study of adolescents initiating DMPA, general measures of diet (energy, carbohydrates, fat, and protein intake) were not predictive of weight gain.[78] However, intake of fiber, magnesium, and linoleic acid were significantly inversely associated with increased BMI over time. All 3 of these nutrients are abundant in foods that benefit overall health. The role of fiber in a healthy diet is well documented.[79] Diets rich in linoleic acid are generally heart healthy.[80,81] Leafy green vegetables, whole grains, nuts, and legumes are good sources of magnesium, which is essential for hundreds of biochemical reactions and physiologic functions.[82] The authors of the study concluded that counseling on diet quality rather than quantity may be more useful for adolescents using DMPA.

Clinical Implications of DMPA-Associated Weight in Adolescents

Risk of DMPA-associated weight gain continues to concern both adolescents and health care professionals. However, weight gain is not a universal finding among adolescents using DMPA. Clinical characteristics, such as race/ethnicity and obesity status, inconsistently predict DMPA-associated weight gain.[83] Early weight gain, defined as more than 5% increase over baseline at 6 months, is currently the best predictor of continued excessive weight gain. Adolescents who have gained 5% or less of baseline weight at 6 months can be reassured that they are unlikely to gain weight on this method. Risks and benefits of continued DMPA use should be weighed carefully in adolescents with early weight gain, including risk of unintended pregnancy with method discontinuation. All adolescents initiating DMPA should be counseled on diet quality.

BLEEDING

Like all progestin-only contraceptives, DMPA can cause changes in menstrual bleeding pattern.[84] Irregular menstrual bleeding is the most common reason cited by adolescents for discontinuing DMPA.[63] As such, it is imperative to counsel all adolescents interested in this contraceptive method to anticipate this change.

Historically, contraceptive trials have not collected standardized data on bleeding and spotting, which has complicated discussion of this adverse effect.[85] However, most adolescents experience some disruption of menstrual bleeding pattern while using DMPA. Altered menstrual bleeding can take a variety of forms, including irregular bleeding or spotting, complete lack of menses, or, rarely, heavy or continuous bleeding. Over time, the frequency of amenorrhea increases, so adolescents can be reassured that bleeding profile tends to improve with subsequent injections. At 12 months, the rate of amenorrhea is reported to be 55% and increases to 68% by 2 years.[86] Despite the increased prevalence of irregular menstrual bleeding among adolescents using DMPA, it is important for health care professionals to be mindful of other causes of menstrual disruption in this population, such as sexually transmitted infections and pregnancy, particularly when irregular bleeding is persistent or severe.[13]

Predictors of Menstrual Pattern During DMPA Use

Little is known regarding predictors of irregular menstrual bleeding pattern on this contraceptive method. Frequency of initial DMPA injections may impact time to amenorrhea. Although early second DMPA injection at 6 weeks was not found to decrease the total number of days of bleeding compared to DMPA at 3-month intervals (14.3 ± 3.7 vs 17.1 ± 4.0; $P = .62$),[72] receipt of monthly DMPA injections for 3 months followed by conversion to 3-month dosing intervals significantly ($P < .001$) reduced time to amenorrhea.[66]

DMPA dose does not seem to affect menstrual pattern. Contraceptive clinical trials in adult women report similar rates of amenorrhea with use of DMPA-SC compared to DMPA-IM.[13,87] In a randomized clinical trial of 3 doses of DMPA IM among adolescents,[48] no significant differences were evident in the number of unscheduled days of bleeding or spotting between participants receiving 150 or 75 mg every 12 weeks for 48 weeks (data not published).

Management of Unscheduled Bleeding

Management of unscheduled bleeding during DMPA use is similar to that for other progestin-only contraceptives. A systematic review conducted in 2013 concluded that additional studies are needed to recommend treatments for vaginal bleeding associated with progestin-only contraception.[88] Despite these limitations, published recommendations for management of this adverse effect are available.[84] It is first important to obtain a detailed description of the bleeding pattern and to distinguish bleeding that is bothersome to the adolescent from that which is tolerable or insignificant. Only the former requires treatment.

Nonsteroidal anti-inflammatory drugs (NSAIDs) are a good first-choice therapy for treatment of bothersome unscheduled bleeding. A randomized placebo-controlled trial of mefenamic acid (500 mg 2 times per day for 5 days) reported a significantly higher percentage of subjects in whom bleeding was stopped during the first week after initial treatment in the mefenamic acid group compared to the placebo group (69.6% vs 40.0%; $P < .05$). However, these effects were not sustained at 4 weeks.[89] A similar trial of the NSAID valdecoxib found it also was effective in the short term.[90] For many women, naproxen may be more readily available and affordable than other NSAIDs. A short trial of naproxen (500 mg 2 times per day for 5 days) can be initiated in patients with no contraindications to NSAID use.[84]

Estrogen is another therapeutic option for bothersome bleeding in adolescents with no estrogen contraindications. Ethinyl estradiol (50 mcg orally daily for 14 days) has previously been shown to successfully stop bleeding in 93% of cases compared to 74% with placebo.[91] As with NSAIDs, however, the effects of estrogen supplementation are not sustained. Because ethinyl estradiol monotherapy is not available in the United States, use of COC daily for 14 days is an acceptable alternative.[84] For some adolescents with persistent bothersome bleeding who enjoy the contraceptive benefits of DMPA, extended COC use can be considered.

Other therapies that have been investigated for treatment of DMPA-associated unscheduled bleeding include doxycycline, tranexamic acid, and mifepristone. Doxycycline (100 mg 2 times per day for 5 days) has not demonstrated benefit.[92] In contrast, tranexamic acid was found to be effective for the short-term treatment of DMPA-associated bleeding. In a clinical trial, 88% of those receiving tranexamic acid (250 mg 4 times per day for 5 days) were bleeding-free during the first week after initial treatment compared to 8.2% of those on placebo

($P < .001$).[93] Four weeks after initial treatment, a bleeding-free interval of more than 20 days was found in 68% of subjects treated with tranexamic acid and 0% treated with placebo ($P < .001$). Mifepristone (50 mg daily for 14 days) has been shown to decrease the incidence of unscheduled bleeding in new starters of DMPA.[94] Studied doses of tranexamic acid and mifepristone are currently not available in the United States.

SUMMARY AND RECOMMENDATIONS

DMPA continues to be an excellent contraceptive choice for adolescents (Table 1). Approximately 1 in 5 adolescent females have used this method. Release of the lower-dose DMPA-SC affords the opportunity for self-

Table 1
Executive summary

Bone mineral density
- For the majority of individuals, BMD values remain in the normal range even after DMPA-associated BMD losses.
- BMD loss is largely reversible after method discontinuation.
- Clinical relevance (ie, fracture risk) of BMD loss has not been established.
- BMD assessment before DMPA initiation can be considered for adolescents with other risk factors for low BMD (eg, low body weight).
- Adequate calcium and vitamin D intake and weight-bearing exercise should be recommended to all adolescents receiving DMPA.

Weight
- Weight gain is not a universal finding among adolescents using DMPA.
- Approximately 1 in 4 adolescents using DMPA is at risk for excessive weight gain.
- Early weight gain (defined as >5% over baseline at 6 months) is the best predictor of continued excessive weight gain.
- Research has not supported increased appetite or caloric intake as the mechanism of DMPA-associated weight gain.
- Counseling for adolescents initiating DMPA should focus on improving overall diet quality (ie, adequate whole grain and vegetable intake).

Bleeding
- Most adolescent experience some change or disruption of menstrual bleeding pattern while using DMPA.
- Frequency of amenorrhea increases with longer duration of use.
- Adolescent must be counseled to anticipate change in bleeding pattern.
- Unscheduled bleeding need only be treated when it is bothersome to the adolescent.
- Short courses of NSAIDs or COC can provide short-term relief of bothersome bleeding.

DMPA dose and formulation
- Contraceptive efficacy is equivalent for 150 mg DMPA-IM and 104 mg DMPA-SC.
- For the most part, the adverse effect profile is similar between the 2 DMPA formulations.
- DMPA-SC has the added benefit of potential for self-administration at home.
- Many adolescents are interested and capable of self-administration of DMPA-SC.
- Wider availability of the DMPA-SC self-administration option is needed for adolescents.

BMD, bone mineral density; COC, combined oral contraceptive; DMPA, depot medroxyprogesterone acetate; IM, intramuscular; NSAID, nonsteroidal anti-inflammatory drug; SC, subcutaneous.

administration at home, but the potential for this therapy has not been fully realized. Health care professionals should work to make the DMPA-SC self-administration option more widely available to their adolescent patients. Patient satisfaction and method continuation can be maximized through (1) appropriate patient screening before DMPA initiation (eg, BMD screening in individuals at high risk for baseline low BMD); (2) comprehensive counseling so that patients can anticipate potential adverse effects (eg, bleeding); and (3) encouragement of healthy lifestyle habits to mitigate adverse effects (ie, high-quality diet, adequate calcium and vitamin D intake, and weight-bearing exercise).

QUESTIONS

1. A 17-year-old patient who initiated depot medroxyprogesterone acetate (DMPA) 24 weeks ago returns for her third injection. She reports that she is very satisfied with the method overall but thinks that she "may have put on a few pounds." She states that she is not dissatisfied with her current weight but is concerned about "a drastic change" if she keeps using DMPA. You review her chart and note that her weight when she initiated DMPA was 122 pounds, and her BMI for age was at the 79th percentile. Her weight today is 127 pounds, and her BMI for age is at the 83rd percentile. You calculate that the patient has gained 4.1% of her baseline weight. How would you counsel this patient about her risk of future weight gain if she continues using DMPA?
   A. Reassure the patient that she was not overweight when she started using DMPA and that she is not overweight now, so she is not at high risk for excessive weight gain.
   B. Reassure the patient that because her 6-month weight gain is no more than 5% of her baseline weight, she is at low risk for continued excessive weight gain while using DMPA.
   C. Reassure the patient that reducing her daily caloric intake will mitigate any future DMPA-associated weight gain.
   D. Reassure the patient that because she has gained less than 10 pounds in 6 months, she is not likely to gain more weight while using DMPA.
2. A 15 year-old-patient returns to your office for a follow-up visit. She started using 104 mg DMPA-SC 6 weeks ago and states that she "loves not having to take a pill every day." When you ask her about adverse effects from the method, she responds that she recently experienced 10 days of "light bleeding" that required use of panty liners. When you ask about sexual activity, she reports that she has not had sex since she broke up with her boyfriend 4 months ago. In reviewing her chart, you note that she received pregnancy and sexually transmitted infection (STI) screening at her DMPA initiation visit. What must you do before prescribing treatment for this patient's report of unscheduled bleeding while using DMPA?

A. Determine whether the patient finds her bleeding pattern bothersome or if it is tolerable.
B. Determine whether an STI is the underlying cause of the patient's bleeding.
C. Determine whether the patient is willing to switch from 104 mg DMPA subcutaneously to 150 mg DMPA intramuscularly.
D. Determine whether the patient would be willing to receive injections on a 6-week dosing interval.

3. A healthy 16-year-old female presents for an annual routine physical examination. The patient has been using DMPA for the past 2 years. She needs contraception and likes DMPA better than the other methods she has tried in the past (combined oral contraceptive and ring). She is not interested in long-acting reversible contraception. She wants to continue using DMPA, but a friend told her that "doctors aren't allowed to give it to you for more than two years." What would be the correct management for this patient?
A. Continue to prescribe DMPA because the 2-year use boxed warning applies only to adults.
B. Continue to prescribe DMPA because adolescence is a category 1 condition according to the U.S. Medical Eligibility Criteria for Contraceptive Use.
C. Continue to prescribe DMPA because you have engaged your patient in a full discussion of risks and benefits.
D. Continue to prescribe DMPA because your patient has agreed to undergo dual-energy X-ray absorptiometry scans twice annually as long as she keeps using DMPA.

(See page 201 for answers.)

References

1. Potts M, Paxman JM. Depo-Provera—ethical issues in its testing and distribution. *J Med Ethics.* 1984;10:9-20
2. Abma JC, Chandra A, Mosher WD, Peterson LS, Piccinino LJ. Fertility, family planning, and women's health: new data from the 1995 National Survey of Family Growth. *Vital Health Stat.* 23 1997:1-114
3. Abma JC, Martinez GM. Sexual activity and contraceptive use among teenagers in the United States, 2011-2015. *Natl Health Stat Report.* 2017;104:1-23
4. Darroch JE, Singh W. *Why Is Teenage Pregnancy Declining? The Roles of Abstinence, Sexual Activity and Contraceptive Use, Occasional Report, No. 1.* New York: The Alan Guttmacher Institute; 1999
5. Nelson A. Merits of DMPA relative to other reversible contraceptive methods. *J Reprod Med.* 2002;47:781-784
6. Potter J, Rubin SE, Sherman P. Fear of intrauterine contraception among adolescents in New York City. *Contraception.* 2014;89:446-450
7. Rose SB, Cooper AJ, Baker NK, Lawton B. Attitudes toward long-acting reversible contraception among young women seeking abortion. *J Womens Health (Larchmt).* 2011;20:1729-1735
8. Okpo E, Allerton L, Brechin S. 'But you can't reverse a hysterectomy!' Perceptions of long acting reversible contraception (LARC) among young women aged 16-24 years: a qualitative study. *Public Health.* 2014;128:934-939

9. Bassol S, Garza-Flores J, Cravioto MC, et al. Ovarian function following a single administration of depo-medroxyprogesterone acetate (DMPA) at different doses. *Fertil Steril.* 1984;42:216-222
10. Kirton KT, Cornette JC. Return of ovulatory cyclicity following an intramuscular injection of medroxyprogesterone acetate (Provera). *Contraception.* 1974;10:39-45
11. Fotherby K, Koetsawang S, Mathrubutham M. Pharmacokinetic study of different doses of Depo Provera. *Contraception.* 1980;22:527-536
12. Said S, Omar K, Koetsawang S, et al. A multicentred phase III comparative clinical trial of depot-medroxyprogesterone acetate given three-monthly at doses of 100 mg or 150 mg: 1. Contraceptive efficacy and side effects. World Health Organization Task Force on Long-Acting Systemic Agents for Fertility Regulation. Special Programme of Research, Development and Research Training in Human Reproduction. *Contraception.* 1986;34:223-235
13. Depo-subQ Provera 104. Physician Information. New York: Pharmacia & UpJohn Company, Division of Pfizer Inc; 2010
14. Jain J, Dutton C, Nicosia A, Wajszczuk C, Bode FR, Mishell DR Jr. Pharmacokinetics, ovulation suppression and return to ovulation following a lower dose subcutaneous formulation of Depo-Provera. *Contraception.* 2004;70:11-18
15. Depo-Provera Contraception Injection. Physician Information. Kalamazoo, MI: Pharmacia & Upjohn Company, a subsidiary of Pharmacia Corporation; 2002
16. Jain J, Jakimiuk AJ, Bode FR, Ross D, Kaunitz AM. Contraceptive efficacy and safety of DMPA-SC. *Contraception.* 2004;70:269-275
17. Williams RL, Hensel DJ, Fortenberry JD. Self-administration of subcutaneous depot medroxyprogesterone acetate by adolescent women. *Contraception.* 2013;88:401-407
18. Cover J, Lim J, Namagembe A, Tumusiime J, Drake JK, Cox CM. Acceptability of Contraceptive Self-Injection with DMPA-SC Among Adolescents in Gulu District, Uganda. *Int Perspect Sex Reprod Health.* 2017;43:153-162
19. Kohn JE, Simons HR, Della Badia L, et al. Increased 1-year continuation of DMPA among women randomized to self-administration: results from a randomized controlled trial at Planned Parenthood. *Contraception.* 2018;97:198-204
20. Sabatier JP, Guaydier-Souquieres G, Benmalek A, Marcelli C. Evolution of lumbar bone mineral content during adolescence and adulthood: a longitudinal study in 395 healthy females 10-24 years of age and 206 premenopausal women. *Osteoporos Int.* 1999;9:476-382
21. Bailey DA, Martin AD, McKay HA, Whiting S, Mirwald R. Calcium accretion in girls and boys during puberty: a longitudinal analysis. *J Bone Miner Res.* 2000;15:2245-2250
22. Bailey DA, McKay HA, Mirwald RL, Crocker PR, Faulkner RA. A six-year longitudinal study of the relationship of physical activity to bone mineral accrual in growing children: the University of Saskatchewan Bone Mineral Accrual Study. *J Bone Miner Res.* 1999;14:1672-1679
23. Slemenda CW, Reister TK, Hui SL, Miller JZ, Christian JC, Johnston CC Jr. Influences on skeletal mineralization in children and adolescents: evidence for varying effects of sexual maturation and physical activity. *J Pediatr.* 1994;125:201-207
24. Henry YM, Fatayerji D, Eastell R. Attainment of peak bone mass at the lumbar spine, femoral neck and radius in men and women: relative contributions of bone size and volumetric bone mineral density. *Osteoporos Int.* 2004;15:263-273
25. Matkovic V, Fontana D, Tominac C, Goel P, Chesnut CH 3rd. Factors that influence peak bone mass formation: a study of calcium balance and the inheritance of bone mass in adolescent females. *Am J Clin Nutr.* 1990;52:878-888
26. Katzman DK, Bachrach LK, Carter DR, Marcus R. Clinical and anthropometric correlates of bone mineral acquisition in healthy adolescent girls. *J Clin Endocrinol Metab.* 1991;73:1332-1339
27. Lu PW, Cowell CT, Lloyd-Jones SA, Briody JN, Howman-Giles R. Volumetric bone mineral density in normal subjects, aged 5-27 years. *J Clin Endocrinol Metab.* 1996;81:1586-1590
28. Bonjour JP, Theintz G, Buchs B, Slosman D, Rizzoli R. Critical years and stages of puberty for spinal and femoral bone mass accumulation during adolescence. *J Clin Endocrinol Metab.* 1991;73:555-563
29. Compston JE. Sex steroids and bone. *Physiol Rev.* 2001;81:419-447

30. Jeppsson S, Johansson. Medroxyprogesterone acetate, estradiol, FSH and LH in peripheral blood after intramuscular administration of Depo-ProveraR to women. *Contraception*. 1976;14:461-469
31. Scholes D, LaCroix AZ, Ichikawa LE, Barlow WE, Ott SM. The association between depot medroxyprogesterone acetate contraception and bone mineral density in adolescent women. *Contraception*. 2004;69:99-104
32. Tharnprisarn W, Taneepanichskul S. Bone mineral density in adolescent and young Thai girls receiving oral contraceptives compared with depot medroxyprogesterone acetate: a cross-sectional study in young Thai women. *Contraception*. 2002;66:101-103
33. Busen NH, Britt RB, Rianon N. Bone mineral density in a cohort of adolescent women using depot medroxyprogesterone acetate for one to two years. *J Adolesc Health*. 2003;32:257-259
34. Cromer BA, Blair JM, Mahan JD, Zibners L, Naumovski Z. A prospective comparison of bone density in adolescent girls receiving depot medroxyprogesterone acetate (Depo-Provera), levonorgestrel (Norplant), or oral contraceptives. *J Pediatr*. 1996;129:671-676
35. Lara-Torre E, Edwards CP, Perlman S, Hertweck SP. Bone mineral density in adolescent females using depot medroxyprogesterone acetate. *J Pediatr Adolesc Gynecol*. 2004;17:17-21
36. Cromer BA, Stager M, Bonny A, et al. Depot medroxyprogesterone acetate, oral contraceptives and bone mineral density in a cohort of adolescent girls. *J Adolesc Health*. 2004;35:434-441
37. Cromer BA, Bonny AE, Stager M, et al. Bone mineral density in adolescent females using injectable or oral contraceptives: a 24-month prospective study. *Fertil Steril*. 2008;90:2060-2067
38. Beksinska ME, Kleinschmidt I, Smit JA, Farley TM. Bone mineral density in a cohort of adolescents during use of norethisterone enanthate, depot-medroxyprogesterone acetate or combined oral contraceptives and after discontinuation of norethisterone enanthate. *Contraception*. 2009;79:345-349
39. Cundy T, Ames R, Horne A, et al. A randomized controlled trial of estrogen replacement therapy in long-term users of depot medroxyprogesterone acetate. *J Clin Endocrinol Metab*. 2003;88:78-81
40. Cromer BA, Lazebnik R, Rome E, et al. Double-blinded randomized controlled trial of estrogen supplementation in adolescent girls who receive depot medroxyprogesterone acetate for contraception. *Am J Obstet Gynecol*. 2005;192:42-47
41. Reid IR. Relationships between fat and bone. *Osteoporos Int*. 2008;19:595-606
42. Gomez-Ambrosi J, Rodriguez A, Catalan V, Fruhbeck G. The bone-adipose axis in obesity and weight loss. *Obes Surg*. 2008;18:1134-1143
43. Leonard MB, Shults J, Wilson BA, Tershakovec AM, Zemel BS. Obesity during childhood and adolescence augments bone mass and bone dimensions. *Am J Clin Nutr*. 2004;80:514-523
44. Bonny AE, Secic M, Cromer BA. Relationship between weight and bone mineral density in adolescents on hormonal contraception. *J Pediatr Adolesc Gynecol*. 2011;24:35-38
45. Harel Z, Johnson CC, Gold MA, et al. Recovery of bone mineral density in adolescents following the use of depot medroxyprogesterone acetate contraceptive injections. *Contraception*. 2010; 81:281-291
46. Committee to Review Dietary Reference Intakes for Vitamin D and Calcium. *DRI Dietary Reference Intakes for Calcium and Vitamin D*. Washington, DC: Nation Academies Press; 2012
47. Kaunitz AM, Darney PD, Ross D, Wolter KD, Speroff L. Subcutaneous DMPA vs. intramuscular DMPA: a 2-year randomized study of contraceptive efficacy and bone mineral density. *Contraception*. 2009;80:7-17
48. Lange HL, Manos BE, Gothard MD, Rogers LK, Bonny AE. Bone mineral density and weight changes in adolescents randomized to 3 doses of depot medroxyprogesterone acetate. *J Pediatr Adolesc Gynecol*. 2017;30:169-175
49. Scholes D, LaCroix AZ, Ichikawa LE, Barlow WE, Ott SM. Change in bone mineral density among adolescent women using and discontinuing depot medroxyprogesterone acetate contraception. *Arch Pediatr Adolesc Med*. 2005;159:139-144
50. Shen C-W, Gaf L, Shang L-H, Wang L-L, Ding H-Q, Jiang H. Effect of depot medroxyprogesterone acetate (DMPA) on bone mineral density (BMD) and evaluating changes in BMD after discontinuation of DMPA in adolescent women. *J Reprod Contracept*. 2015;26:151-159

51. Harel Z, Wolter K, Gold MA, et al. Biopsychosocial variables associated with substantial bone mineral density loss during the use of depot medroxyprogesterone acetate in adolescents: adolescents who lost 5% or more from baseline vs. those who lost less than 5%. *Contraception.* 2010;82:503-512
52. Black Box Warning Added Concerning Long-Term Use of Depo-Provera Contraception Injection. Rockville, MD: US Food and Drug Administration; 2005
53. Hui SL, Slemenda CW, Johnston CC Jr. Age and bone mass as predictors of fracture in a prospective study. *J Clin Invest.* 1988;81:1804-1809
54. Kaunitz AM, Grimes DA. Remove the black-box warning for depot medroxyprogesterone acetate! *OBG Manag.* 2011;23:6-9
55. Cromer BA, Scholes D, Berenson A, et al; Society for Adolescent Medicine. Depot medroxyprogesterone acetate and bone mineral density in adolescents—the Black Box Warning: a Position Paper of the Society for Adolescent Medicine. *J Adolesc Health.* 2006;39:296-301
56. Committee Opinion No. 602: Depot Medroxyprogesterone Acetate and Bone Effects. *Obstet Gynecol.* 2014;123:1398-1402
57. Curtis KM, Tepper NK, Jatlaoui TC, et al. U.S. Medical Eligibility Criteria for Contraceptive Use, 2016. *MMWR Recomm Rep.* 2016;65:1-103
58. O'Dell CM, Forke CM, Polaneczky MM, Sondheimer SJ, Slap GB. Depot medroxyprogesterone acetate or oral contraception in postpartum adolescents. *Obstet Gynecol.* 1998;91:609-614
59. Risser WL, Gefter LR, Barratt MS, Risser JM. Weight change in adolescents who used hormonal contraception. *J Adolesc Health.* 1999;24:433-436
60. Mangan SA, Larsen PG, Hudson S. Overweight teens at increased risk for weight gain while using depot medroxyprogesterone acetate. *J Pediatr Adolesc Gynecol.* 2002;15:79-82
61. Le YC, Rahman M, Berenson AB. Early weight gain predicting later weight gain among depot medroxyprogesterone acetate users. *Obstet Gynecol.* 2009;114:279-284
62. Bonny A, Secic M, Cromer B. Early weight gain related to later weight gain in adolescents on depot medroxyprogesterone acetate. *Obstet Gynecol.* 2011;117:793-797
63. Harel Z, Biro FM, Kollar LM, Rauh JL. Adolescents' reasons for and experience after discontinuation of the long-acting contraceptives Depo-Provera and Norplant. *J Adolesc Health.* 1996;19: 118-123
64. Polaneczky M, Liblanc M. Long-term depot medroxyprogesterone acetate (Depo-Provera) use in inner-city adolescents. *J Adolesc Health.* 1998;23:81-88
65. Moore LL, Valuck R, McDougall C, Fink W. A comparative study of one-year weight gain among users of medroxyprogesterone acetate, levonorgestrel implants, and oral contraceptives. *Contraception.* 1995;52:215-219
66. Templeman C, Boyd H, Hertweck SP. Depomedroxyprogesterone acetate use and weight gain among adolescents. *J Pediatr Adolesc Gynecol.* 2000;13:45-46
67. Lopez LM, Ramesh S, Chen M, et al. Progestin-only contraceptives: effects on weight. *Cochrane Database Syst Rev.* 2016;8:CD008815
68. Bonny A, Camlin K, Harvey R, Islam K, Debanne S, Cromer B. Prospective analysis of weight changes in adolescent females initiating depot medroxyprogesterone acetate (DMPA), oral contraceptive pills (OC), or no hormonal contraceptive method (abstract). *J Adolesc Health.* 2003; 32:134
69. Berenson AB, Rahman M. Changes in weight, total fat, percent body fat, and central-to-peripheral fat ratio associated with injectable and oral contraceptive use. *Am J Obstet Gynecol.* 2009;200: 329.e1-e8
70. Bonny AE, Britto MT, Huang B, Succop P, Slap GB. Weight gain, adiposity, and eating behaviors among adolescent females on depot medroxyprogesterone acetate (DMPA). *J Pediatr Adolesc Gynecol.* 2004;17:109-115
71. Bonny AE, Lange HL, Hade EM, Kaufman B, Reed MD, Mesiano S. Serum adipocytokines and adipose weight gain: a pilot study in adolescent females initiating depot medroxyprogesterone acetate. *Contraception.* 2015;92:298-300

72. Harel Z, Biro FM, Kollar LM. Depo-Provera in adolescents: effects of early second injection or prior oral contraception. *J Adolesc Health*. 1995;16:379-384
73. Bonny AE, Lange HL, Rogers LK, Gothard DM, Reed MD. A pilot study of depot medroxyprogesterone acetate pharmacokinetics and weight gain in adolescent females. *Contraception*. 2014;89: 357-360
74. Clark MK, Dillon JS, Sowers M, Nichols S. Weight, fat mass, and central distribution of fat increase when women use depot-medroxyprogesterone acetate for contraception. *Int J Obes*. 2005;29: 1252-1258
75. Dal'Ava N, Bahamondes L, Bahamondes MV, Bottura BF, Monteiro I. Body weight and body composition of depot medroxyprogesterone acetate users. *Contraception*. 2014;90:182-187
76. Bonny AE, Secic M, Cromer BA. A longitudinal comparison of body composition changes in adolescent girls receiving hormonal contraception. *J Adolesc Health*. 2009;45:423-425
77. Amatayakul K, Sivasomboon B, Thanangkul O. A study of the mechanism of weight gain in medroxyprogesterone acetate users. *Contraception*. 1980;22:605-622
78. Lange HL, Belury MA, Secic M, Thomas A, Bonny AE. Dietary intake and weight gain among adolescents on depot medroxyprogesterone acetate. *J Pediatr Adolesc Gynecol*. 2015;28:139-143
79. Anderson JW, Baird P, Davis RH Jr, et al. Health benefits of dietary fiber. *Nutr Rev*. 2009;67: 188-205
80. Norris LE, Collene AL, Asp ML, et al. Comparison of dietary conjugated linoleic acid with safflower oil on body composition in obese postmenopausal women with type 2 diabetes mellitus. *Am J Clin Nutr*. 2009;90:468-476
81. Czernichow S, Thomas D, Bruckert E. n-6 Fatty acids and cardiovascular health: a review of the evidence for dietary intake recommendations. *Br J Nutr*. 2010;104:788-796
82. Vormann J. Magnesium: nutrition and metabolism. *Mol Aspects Med*. 2003;24:27-37
83. Gerlach LS, Saldaña SN, Wang Y, Nick TG, Spigarelli MG. Retrospective review of the relationship between weight change and demographic factors following initial depot medroxyprogesterone acetate injection in adolescents. *Clin Ther*. 2011;33:182-187
84. Zigler RE, McNicholas C. Unscheduled vaginal bleeding with progestin-only contraceptive use. *Am J Obstet Gynecol*. 2017;216:443-450
85. Mishell DR Jr, Guillebaud J, Westhoff C, et al. Recommendations for standardization of data collection and analysis of bleeding in combined hormone contraceptive trials. *Contraception*. 2007;75:11-15
86. Schwallie PC, Assenzo JR. Contraceptive use—efficacy study utilizing medroxyprogesterone acetate administered as an intramuscular injection once every 90 days. *Fertil Steril*. 1973;24:331-339
87. Arias RD, Jain JK, Brucker C, Ross D, Ray A. Changes in bleeding patterns with depot medroxyprogesterone acetate subcutaneous injection 104 mg. *Contraception*. 2006;74:234-238
88. Abdel-Aleem H, d'Arcangues C, Vogelsong KM, Gaffield ML, Gulmezoglu AM. Treatment of vaginal bleeding irregularities induced by progestin only contraceptives. *Cochrane Database Syst Rev*. 2013;7:Cd003449
89. Tantiwattanakul P, Taneepanichskul S. Effect of mefenamic acid on controlling irregular uterine bleeding in DMPA users. *Contraception*. 2004;70:277-279
90. Nathirojanakun P, Taneepanichskul S, Sappakitkumjorn N. Efficacy of a selective COX-2 inhibitor for controlling irregular uterine bleeding in DMPA users. *Contraception*. 2006;73:584-587
91. Said S, Sadek W, Rocca M, et al. Clinical evaluation of the therapeutic effectiveness of ethinyl oestradiol and oestrone sulphate on prolonged bleeding in women using depot medroxyprogesterone acetate for contraception. World Health Organization, Special Programme of Research, Development and Research Training in Human Reproduction, Task Force on Long-acting Systemic Agents for Fertility Regulation. *Hum Reprod*. 1996;11(Suppl 2):1-13

92. Abdel-Aleem H, Shaaban OM, Abdel-Aleem MA, Fetih GN. Doxycycline in the treatment of bleeding with DMPA: a double-blinded randomized controlled trial. *Contraception*. 2012;86: 224-230
93. Senthong AJ, Taneepanichskul S. The effect of tranexamic acid for treatment irregular uterine bleeding secondary to DMPA use. *J Med Assoc Thai*. 2009;92:461-465
94. Jain JK, Nicosia AF, Nucatola DL, Lu JJ, Kuo J, Felix JC. Mifepristone for the prevention of breakthrough bleeding in new starters of depo-medroxyprogesterone acetate. *Steroids*. 2003;68:1115-1119

Adolesc Med 030 (2019) 102–117

Intrauterine Devices for Adolescents: Guidance for Clinicians

Andrea J. Hoopes, MD, MPH[a*]; Gina S. Sucato, MD, MPH[b]

[a]Adolescent Center, Washington Permanente Medical Group, Seattle, Washington; [b]Director, Adolescent Center, Washington Permanente Medical Group, Adjunct Investigator, Kaiser Permanente Washington Health Research Institute, Seattle, Washington

LEARNING OBJECTIVES

After reviewing this article, the reader should be able to:

1. Describe the indications and contraindications for intrauterine contraception in adolescent patients
2. Improve skills in preinsertion counseling and anticipatory guidance for intrauterine contraception in adolescent patients
3. Recognize potential barriers to adolescents initiating intrauterine contraception and potential solutions to address these barriers

BACKGROUND

Intrauterine devices (IUDs) are contraceptive devices placed within the uterus. The primary mechanism of action of both copper and levonorgestrel-releasing IUDs is prevention of fertilization by impairing sperm function and viability.[1,2] The levonorgestrel IUDs also thicken cervical mucus and suppress the uterine lining.[3,4] The available evidence supports that IUDs do not disrupt pregnancy,[5] which begins with implantation of a fertilized egg.[6]

This article will describe the current evidence base for evaluating an adolescent patient for intrauterine contraception, adolescent-centered counseling and placement principles, and key management strategies for potential side effects and complications. The article concludes with a discussion of unique challenges regarding IUD use by adolescents and potential solutions.

---

*Corresponding author
E-mail address: Andrea.J1.Hoopes@kp.org

 ISSN 1934-4287

Historically, adolescents were not considered to be appropriate candidates for IUDs, mostly based on nulliparous status and now disproven concerns for detrimental effects on fertility, as well as concerns that the high rates of sexually transmitted infections (STIs) among adolescents could lead to an increase in complications. However, in 2007, the American College of Obstetrics and Gynecology (ACOG) published a committee opinion informed by a growing body of evidence supporting the safety of IUDs for adolescent patients.[7] Currently both ACOG and the American Academy of Pediatrics (AAP) consider IUDs first-line contraceptive options for adolescents.[8,9] In the past decade, initiatives to promote adolescent access to IUD services have grown as the medical and public health communities have acknowledged the immense potential of IUDs to contribute significantly to teen pregnancy prevention efforts. Furthermore, IUDs have emerged as valuable medical treatment of gynecologic conditions in many populations, including young women with physical or cognitive disabilities; transgender, non-binary, and gender-diverse youth seeking menstrual suppression or contraception; and adolescents who have previously experienced pregnancy and are at risk for rapid repeat pregnancy.

ASSESSING FOR ELIGIBILITY

As awareness and demand for IUDs increase, clinicians must be able to rapidly assess whether a patient may be an appropriate candidate for IUD placement. As discussed in the article on adolescent pregnancy prevention and application of Centers for Disease Control and Prevention (CDC) evidence-based contraception guidance by Zapata et al in this issue of AM:STARs, the CDC U.S. Medical Eligibility Criteria for Contraceptive Use (US MEC) provides evidence-based guidance to assist physicians and other clinicians in establishing eligibility.[10] With regard to age, adolescents who have achieved menarche but are younger than 20 years are considered a US MEC category 2 for initiation and continuation of copper and levonorgestrel IUDs (ie, advantages generally outweigh theoretical or proven risks and method can be used). The US MEC notes that concern exists about risk for both expulsion from nulliparous uteri and STI from sexual behavior in younger age groups.[10] A systematic review conducted for the most recent US MEC update included 11 studies of variable quality comparing the outcome of expulsion among younger versus older women. The authors found that the majority of studies suggested a decreasing risk of expulsion with increasing age for copper IUDs, with mixed results for levonorgestrel IUDs.[11] The review also explored risk of infection with IUD use among young women, noting that the existing studies are challenged by use of inappropriate comparison groups, overdiagnosis of pelvic inflammatory disease (PID) among IUD users, and failure to control for confounders such as sexual behavior or condom use. The highest-quality evidence did not find any difference in PID rates among young women using IUDs compared to those using other methods.[11] Evidence-based guidance from ACOG, AAP, the CDC, and the Society of Family Planning all support the safety of IUDs for adolescents.[8-10,12]

The few absolute contraindications for IUD use in women of all ages include current purulent cervicitis or known chlamydial or gonococcal infection, current PID, anatomic uterine abnormalities distorting the uterine cavity in a manner incompatible with IUD insertion, unexplained vaginal bleeding (before evaluation), and, for the levonorgestrel IUD, current breast cancer. Those with malignant hepatomas or history of breast cancer in the past with no evidence of disease for 5 years are US MEC category 3 (ie, theoretical or proven risks generally outweigh advantages and method should not be used unless no other alternatives exist).

COUNSELING PRINCIPLES

The counseling needs of adolescents seeking contraception are complex and highly variable based on developmental stage, personal past experience with contraception, and social support systems.[13-15] Thus, clinicians should assess whether adolescents have adequate cognitive capacity to provide informed consent for the procedure and to seek care for potential side effects and complications should they arise. A trusted adult who can facilitate follow-up needs that may occur should also be identified. Establishing the patient's baseline level of understanding about anatomy and how pregnancy occurs can guide the possible need for visual aids, uterine models, and multimedia resources to ensure adequate transfer of knowledge. Although an efficacy-based counseling strategy has been supported in adolescent and adult patients,[16] no standard counseling approaches specific to adolescent patients have been established and validated. The current standard is informed largely by qualitative studies that explore common concerns and decision-making factors identified in adolescent patients. These include fear of pain during the procedure, discomfort with the idea of having something "placed" inside of them, concern about risk for perforation and other complications, and a desire to avoid unpredictable bleeding patterns.[17-20] In addition to managing individualized concerns, standard preinsertion counseling messages include an explanation of the known risks and benefits of intrauterine contraception. Established rates of perforation are low (<1 per 1000 insertions),[21] whereas expulsion rates over time can range from 3% to 20% for adolescents.[8,22-25] A discussion of benefits can include the very low contraceptive failure rate (<1%) as well as a range of non-contraceptive benefits, including, for some IUD users, lighter periods or complete menstrual suppression, management of dysmenorrhea, method privacy, and no need for refills or other recurrent treatments once the IUD is in place.

In the United States, 2 types of IUDs are available, hormonal and non-hormonal. The copper T is the only non-hormonal IUD option available in the United States. The copper T380-A IUD (ParaGard; Teva North America, North Wales, PA) is approved for 10 years of use but has been shown to be effective for 12 years.[26] It has a failure rate of 0.8% with typical method use.[27] The failure rate with typical method use describes the percentage of women who experience an accidental pregnancy during the first year if they do not stop use for any other reason. Hormonal (levonorgestrel-containing) IUDs are also very effective, with typical use failure rates of less than 0.2%.[27] Four hormonal IUDs are currently approved in the United States and differ primarily by the amount of levonorgestrel: Liletta (52-mg levonorgestrel; Medicines360, San Francisco, CA; and Allergan, Dublin, Ireland); Mirena (52-mg levonorgestrel; Bayer HealthCare Pharmaceuticals Inc, Wayne NJ); Kyleena (19.5-mg levonorgestrel; Bayer HealthCare Pharmaceuticals); and Skyla (13.5-mg levonorgestrel (Bayer HealthCare Pharmaceuticals). These levonorgestrel IUDs are approved for 3 (Skyla) to 5 (Kyleena, Liletta, Mirena) years of use, although a 52-mg levonorgestrel device has been found to safely prevent pregnancy for up to 7 years.[28] Although only Skyla has been approved by the US Food and Drug Administration for use in adolescents younger than 18, the CDC US MEC supports placing any intrauterine device available in the United States in a postmenarchal adolescent patient. Cost may be a consideration, and often clinics may stock only certain types of IUDs.

PLACEMENT OF IUDs

Placement of an IUD on the same day it is requested by the patient is considered best practice, as long as the clinician can be reasonably certain the patient is not pregnant and that there are sufficient assurances that the adolescent does not feel coerced into a procedure without adequate considerations of personal preferences. If same-day placement is not feasible, patients need a clear follow-up plan with instructions to minimize risk for pregnancy in the interim and to ensure no additional barriers to care arise. Although some clinicians have more success with placement during menstrual bleeding, IUDs can be inserted at any time during the menstrual cycle if it is reasonably certain that woman is not pregnant. Of note, the copper IUD can be used for emergency contraception within 5 days of unprotected sexual intercourse. Ongoing studies, such as this randomized controlled trial (https://clinicaltrials.gov/ct2/show/NCT01539720) are currently underway to test the levonorgestrel IUD as a potential method for emergency contraception.

Placement procedure begins with informed consent and ascertaining that the patient is not pregnant. Most clinicians will perform a urine pregnancy test before any IUD placement regardless of current contraceptive method. Standard equipment is outlined in Table 1, although individual clinician practices vary.

The procedure begins with a focused physical examination, including measuring vital signs, assessing for adequate hydration, and performing an abdominal examination and bimanual examination to determine the position of the uterus and to assess for any evidence of uterine, adnexal, or cervical motion tenderness. The patient remains in the supine position in stirrups for the remainder of the procedure. The clinicians should initially assess for any vulvovaginal lesions, vaginal discharge, or marked inguinal lymphadenopathy that may raise suspi-

Table 1
Equipment for IUD placement

Adjustable examination table with stirrups
Speculum with adequate lighting
Betadine or chlorhexidine (confirm that patient is not allergic or cross allergic)
Large cotton swabs
Swab for nucleic acid amplification testing for *Neisseria gonorrhoeae* and *Chlamydia trachomatis* (if not performed on urine)
Tenaculum
Uterine sound[a]
Package containing IUD and inserter
Gloves for examination and sterile gloves for IUD placement
Lubricant for bimanual examination
Scissors
Disposable underpads (Chux pads)
Sanitary pad for patient
Heat pack
Optional: dilators, lidocaine and paracervical block needle, ferric subsulfate solution or silver nitrate for hemostasis, ibuprofen, ringed forceps for removal

IUD, intrauterine device.
[a] Some experts believe that risk for perforation may be lower with plastic sounds than with metal sounds.

cion for genital infection. If a woman has not been screened for STIs according to STI screening guidelines,[29] screening can be performed at the time of insertion.

For many adolescents, IUD insertion may be their first experience with an examination using a speculum, and standard efforts to increase comfort should be used, such as warming the speculum, moistening it with water or lubricant, and, if needed, inserting it over a finger providing downward pressure. Occasionally a patient will prefer to insert the speculum herself with clinician guidance, particularly if there is a history of trauma or a previous negative experience with a pelvic examination. Special consideration should be taken when counseling about and placing IUDs in transgender or gender non-binary youth who may face additional barriers to comfort with pelvic examinations. Having everything needed for the IUD insertion set up in advance and minimizing the time the speculum is in place can decrease discomfort.

Upon speculum placement, the clinician should ensure that the cervical os is clearly visualized and there is no evidence of purulent cervicitis or other gross cervical abnormality. The cervix is cleaned using povidone-iodine (Betadine) or chlorhexidine, then a tenaculum is placed at 12 o'clock for an anteverted or mid-position uterus or 6 o'clock for a retroverted uterus. Tension on the tenaculum is applied and a uterine sound is introduced, ensuring a depth of at least 6 cm required for IUD placement. The IUD package is opened, the IUD loaded, the inserter prepared according to the measured depth of the uterus, and the IUD placed according to individual inserter instructions. Details on individual placement techniques for the different types of IUDs and inserters are beyond the scope of this chapter. When the tenaculum is removed, adequate hemostasis should be assured, providing pressure with a large cotton swab if needed. Strings should then be trimmed to 3 to 4 cm, taking care not to pull on the strings when withdrawing the scissors, and the speculum removed. Patients should be monitored by a health care practitioner until they feel well enough to ambulate without dizziness or discomfort.

PAIN MANAGEMENT

One of the barriers to an adolescent obtaining an IUD is the perception that insertion will be painful.[19,30-32] Younger patients are at increased risk for pain with IUD insertion, particularly if they are nulliparous or have a history of anxiety or dysmenorrhea.[33] Given that high levels of anticipated pain correlate with high levels of experienced pain during IUD insertion,[33] clinicians should strive to minimize preinsertion expectation of pain. While acknowledging that some degree of discomfort is common during placement, some experts believe that carefully chosen language may be helpful, for example, avoiding words such as *pain* and *pinch*, which may heighten the anticipation of pain. Additionally, it may be calming for patients to use self-chosen distractions, such as watching videos or listening to music. Having a friend or family member in the room can be helpful, provided that person is comfortable being present during the procedure and is unlikely to escalate patient anxiety. However, if available, an additional member of the health care team, such as a medical assistant, may be a more reliable source of reassurance and distraction.[34] The clinician should ask and honor patient preferences regarding how much description they would like of exactly what the clinician is doing in real time.

Topical, locally injected, and systemic medications to minimize discomfort during IUD placement have all been studied. Pain with IUD placement is decreased with topical lidocaine-prilocaine cream, topical lidocaine 4% gel in nulliparous women, and 10% lidocaine spray in parous women.[35] Although topical 2% lidocaine gel has not been found to decrease pain with IUD placement,[35] 1 study found it helpful during placement of the tenaculum in nulliparous women.[36] Patient sensation of tenaculum placement may be diminished by placing it slowly, which will also soften the jarring noise as it clicks into position. A paracervical block with 1% lidocaine has been shown to decrease pain with tenaculum placement and with insertion specifically in nulliparous adolescents and young adults.[37] However, overall satisfaction with the IUD insertion procedure in this study did not differ. Given the increased time, expense, and potential side effects associated with paracervical blocks (eg, metallic taste, tinnitus, or patient-reported cardiac arrhythmia), they should be used judiciously.

Although ibuprofen is commonly recommended to help with pain after insertion,[38] studies of ibuprofen in doses of 400 to 800 mg before IUD placement have not been shown to decrease pain during insertion.[35] In parous women, naproxen 550 mg given 1 hour before the procedure relieves insertion pain better than placebo, but not as well as tramadol.[35] However, tramadol has been classified as a controlled substance (class 4) since 2014. Ketorolac 30 mg intramuscularly decreases pain after (but not during) placement.[39] Oral Ketorolac 20 mg is moderately effective in decreasing pain during and after IUD placement when given 40 to 60 minutes before the procedure in women older than 18 years and at least 50 kg in weight.[40]

One randomized controlled trial has found misoprostol 200 mcg given vaginally 10 hours and 4 hours before insertion is useful in second attempts of a previously failed insertion (87.5% vs 61.9%).[41] However, misoprostol should not be given routinely for IUD insertion, as studies have found it does not minimize pain but does increase side effects, such as nausea, diarrhea, and abdominal cramping.[35,42]

General anesthesia for IUD placement may be considered for certain adolescent patients, including those with developmental delay or those who had previous placement attempts that were unsuccessful without sedation.[43] In these rare circumstances, clinicians, patients, and caregivers should reach consensus that the risks associated with general anesthesia are outweighed by the potential benefits of intrauterine contraception and the procedure could not be feasibly performed without anesthesia.[34]

FOLLOW-UP

After a successful IUD placement, clear verbal and written instructions should be provided, including information about the time interval required for effective contraception with the IUD (7 days for levonorgestrel IUD, thus requiring a backup method; immediately for the copper IUD.) Patients should be advised not to place anything in the vagina for 7 days. Teens may require explicit instructions regarding avoiding tampons, insertive sex, and checking for strings during this time. Ultrasound confirmation of placement is not routinely performed unless there are concerns about severe pain during or after the procedure, heavy bleeding, or unrecognized expulsion.[44]

Routine follow-up is not necessary, although many clinicians find that teens benefit from scheduled follow-up in 4 to 6 weeks to assess for any side effects, satisfaction, and provide anticipatory guidance if needed. Many adolescents require additional reassurance about the common experiences of unpredictable bleeding (see section on Complications and Side Effects). Teens should also be counseled about the signs and symptoms of expulsion or partial expulsion, including sudden change in bleeding patterns, pain, palpable components of the device at the cervical os, or discomfort during sex.

Teens should be advised to return any time they want to discuss side effects or other problems, want to change their method, or when it is time to remove or replace the IUD. Any clinician who sees IUD users for reproductive or preventive care should assess the teen's satisfaction with the method, ask about any changes in health status that would change the appropriateness for IUD use, consider performing an examination to check for the presence of strings annually and whenever indicated based on symptoms of expulsion noted earlier, provide counseling regarding condom use for STI prevention, and perform routine testing and treatment of STIs as indicated by the teen's sexual health behaviors.

COMPLICATIONS AND SIDE EFFECTS

Abrupt onset of pain or change in bleeding patterns should prompt the clinician to rule out perforation or expulsion with clinical examination and, when indicated, imaging. Although IUD removal may be required in the event of intolerable pain or irregular bleeding, the presence of PID does not warrant immediate IUD removal. Patients with PID should be treated according to CDC sexually transmitted disease treatment guidelines and carefully reassessed in 48 to 72 hours.[29] If no clinical improvement is seen, antibiotics should be continued and removal of the IUD considered.

If a patient is found to be pregnant after IUD placement, a balanced discussion of comprehensive pregnancy options should take place and patient should be referred to an obstetrics clinician who can offer care according to the patient's preferences and acute needs. If desired, removal of IUD upon diagnosis of pregnancy may be feasible under the care of an expert, depending on the IUD position and estimated gestational age.

Irregular bleeding is sufficiently common during the first 3 to 6 months of IUD use that adolescents should be counseled to expect it and reassured that it is not harmful. However, if a change occurs in a previously stable pattern of bleeding, it is advisable to look for potential explanations such as pregnancy, STI, or IUD displacement.[45]

Anticipatory guidance about bleeding differs by IUD type, as initial bleeding changes are more likely to include heavier bleeding with copper IUDs than hormonal IUDs. A study of 826 copper IUD users and 3001 hormonal IUD users found that more than 70% of copper IUD users experienced heavier bleeding at 3 months compared to baseline, 8% reported lighter bleeding, and 10% reported reduced frequency of bleeding.[46] In comparison, among the hormonal IUD users, fewer than 15% reported heavier bleeding, whereas 67% reported lighter bleeding, and almost half reported reduced frequency of bleeding. At 6-month follow-up, 72% of copper IUD users reported no additional changes in bleeding frequency, whereas 55% of hormonal IUD users reported further decreases in frequency.[46] Consistent with this finding, a study of 256 women using the 52-mg levonorgestrel IUD found that 44% reported amenorrhea after 6 months of use, and that this rate remained stable, with 50% having amenorrhea after 12 and 24 months of use.[47] Oligomenorrhea, defined as scanty bleeding occurring in intervals of every 45 days or longer, was present in an additional one-fourth of women throughout the first 2 years of use. Lower rates of amenorrhea, 20% in the first year of use, are reported by the package insert for this same 52-mg IUD[48] and an even lower level of 6% for the 13.5-mg levonorgestrel IUD.[49]

A systematic review of the treatment of bleeding irregularities in women using copper IUDs found support for use of a variety of nonsteroidal anti-inflammatory drugs to reduce menstrual bleeding for a current bleeding episode and possibly to prevent heavy or prolonged menstrual bleeding.[50] Consistent with this, the US Selected Practice Recommendations for Contraceptive Use recommends short-term treatment with nonsteroidal anti-inflammatory drugs for 5 to 7 days in this scenario.[45] This article did not identify any studies evaluating treatments of bleeding irregularities with levonorgestrel IUD use. However, some clinicians will try a short course of combined hormonal contraceptive pills for 1 to 3 months if patients would like to try this rather than removing their IUD.[51]

CHALLENGES TO IUD USE AMONG ADOLESCENTS

Unique challenges regarding the use of IUDs in adolescents range from barriers to acceptability and uptake of IUDs, to barriers to continuation and removal. Additionally, IUD use in adolescents may present ethical considerations, such as potential for coercion, warranting individualized approach to care.

The historic concerns that adolescents are not appropriate candidates for IUDs have led to challenges in adolescents being consistently offered and supported in choosing IUDs. Despite efforts to increase awareness through web-based initiatives such as bedsider.org and stayteen.org, teens may not be aware of IUDs as an option unless raised by a clinician.[52-56] As in adult women,[57] IUDs are underutilized in teens, and their use remains low relative to shorter-acting methods such as condoms and oral contraceptives. The most comprehensive data from the National Survey for Family Growth found that among adolescents 15 to 19 years old, IUD use increased from 2.5% in 2006 to 2010 to 2.8% in 2011 to 2015.[58] Similarly, among females aged 15 to 19 years seeking contraceptive services in Title X family planning settings from 2005 to 2013, 2.8% were found to have chosen an IUD.[59]

Studies have found that having a friend or family member who likes their own IUD is one of the strongest predictors of IUD uptake among 14-to 24-year-olds.[60] Among adolescents, older age and parity predicted IUD uptake in the Contraceptive CHOICE Project of women accessing no-cost contraceptive options in St. Louis.[61] Consistent with this, nulliparity and having a friend or family member who disliked the method have been associated with low personal acceptability of IUDs.[62] Efforts to address low acceptability of IUDs using brief, clinic-based educational sessions targeting knowledge and acceptability of IUDs have shown promising results.[53] Additionally, the online contraception support network bedsider.org has been shown to increase knowledge and familiarity with contraceptive methods, including IUDs.[63] A large intervention to reduce the cost and access barriers to IUD uptake and to provide standardized counseling presenting methods in order of effectiveness showed IUD uptake of 58% among adolescent patients.[61,64] This intervention, which also resulted in a high uptake of the contraceptive implant, demonstrated a decrease in teen pregnancy rates in the community in which the initiative took place.[65] Similar initiatives in Colorado have also shown dramatic increases in IUD uptake and associated decreases in unplanned pregnancies among adolescents.[66]

An additional challenge is the limited number of health care practitioners who offer IUD services to teens. Several studies have shown that pediatric health care practitioners have variable knowledge about IUD use in teens and may have concerns about providing IUD services because of lack of training, worries about future fertility, parental resistance, and legal consequences.[67-70] Counseling about IUDs and providing IUD services can be hindered by inadequate knowledge, limited opportunities and time constraints, and lack of motivation among clinicians.[71,72] Potential solutions to the challenges of clinician training include the development of a curriculum to provide both didactic and hands-on training in provision of long-acting reversible contraceptives for adolescent medicine rotations and programs, standardizing training in counseling and provision of long-acting reversible contraceptives in adolescent medicine and as an option in pediatric residency programs, and improving collaborations between adolescent medicine and family medicine/obstetrics and gynecology services to allow for colocation of services and cross-training.[73] Additionally, health system-level initiatives such as those pioneered by Upstream USA have the potential to build capacity for IUD services for individuals of all ages, including adolescents.[74,75]

A number of school-based health centers have expanded their contraceptive services and have shown success, with marked increases in adolescents choosing IUDs. This requires a clinician champion, practitioner training, a strategy to obtain institutional support (eg, focusing on IUDs as an opportunity to decrease teen pregnancy rates and therefore increase graduation rates), a focus on IUD safety, clear management protocols, and a supportive community.[76]

Parental concerns about contraceptive methods requiring a medical procedure may present a barrier. Additionally, teens may not be able to obtain parental consent for procedures in states in which it is required, or they may be hesitant to seek services if they know their parent or guardian is not supportive of intrauterine contraception. Engaging parents proactively in discussions about the safety and efficacy of intrauterine contraception during preventive care visits may increase acceptability among adults who care for teens.[77]

Barriers to IUD continuation in adolescents may include intolerable side effects, a desire for pregnancy, or potentially reproductive coercion from a partner who desires pregnancy. Younger age alone has not been shown to be a predictor of early discontinuation of IUDs.[78] Establishing trust in the patient-clinician relationship so that the participants can engage in balanced, patient-centered discussions about the patient's short- and long-term reproductive life plan and feasibility of alternative contraceptive options is essential to ensure that the patient maintains bodily autonomy. A clinician should never refuse to remove an IUD when requested by a patient; however, if side effects are manageable without removal, these options should be presented to the patient.

It must be recognized that adolescents are vulnerable to coercive placement or removal of the device by clinicians, parents, or partners. A reproductive justice framework (ie, one that upholds the human right to maintain personal bodily autonomy, have children, not have children, and parent children in safe and sustainable communities) must be applied to IUD service delivery for all women, but particularly adolescents.[79] Removal should include a discussion of pregnancy intentions. If pregnancy is desired, appropriate preconception counseling should take place; if not, then a plan for an alternative method of contraception should occur.

CONCLUSION

Whenever possible, adolescents should be engaged in program development and research regarding IUD services. Further investigation is needed to delineate standardized, evidence-based counseling strategies that are linked to patient satisfaction and positive outcomes. Additional research gaps include improving the ease, comfort, and success of IUD insertion; timing for safe IUD insertion after pelvic or cervical infection; and managing changes between methods of hormonal contraception and an IUD.[80] An article by Torres and Alderman in this issue of AM:STARs addresses emerging technologies specific to intrauterine contraception, including novel IUDs designed to minimize irregular bleeding and discomfort with procedure.

In summary, IUDs are a safe, highly acceptable, effective method for many adolescents. Special considerations specific to unique populations of adolescents, counseling needs tailored to developmental stage and support systems, adolescent-centered placement and follow-up procedures, and a reproductive justice framework are paramount to high-quality IUD service delivery.

QUESTIONS

1. All of the following are considered absolute contraindications to intrauterine device (IUD) placement except:
   A. Current purulent cervicitis
   B. Age younger than 13 years
   C. Current pelvic inflammatory disease
   D. Current breast cancer for the levonorgestrel IUD
2. Before IUD placement, adolescents should be counseled (choose one):
   A. IUDs and oral contraceptive pills are equally effective in preventing pregnancy.
   B. An IUD must be left in place for 6 months before it can be removed.
   C. Most IUD users have more menstrual bleeding 1 year after insertion than at baseline.
   D. Typical-use failure rates of IUDs are less than 1%.
3. Important considerations related to IUD placement include (choose one):
   A. IUD expulsion is exceptionally rare and occurs only if it is improperly inserted.
   B. The levonorgestrel IUD is approved by the Food and Drug Administration for emergency contraception for up to 7 days after unprotected sexual intercourse.
   C. In asymptomatic women, screening for sexually transmitted infection can be performed on the same day as IUD insertion.
   D. Lidocaine is ineffective in reducing pain associated with IUD insertion unless it is provided via paracervical block.

(See page 202 for answers.)

References

1. Patai K, Szilagyi G, Noszal B, Szentmariay I. Local tissue effects of copper-containing intrauterine devices. *Fertil Steril.* 2003;80(5):1281-1283
2. Ortiz ME, Croxatto HB. Copper-T intrauterine device and levonorgestrel intrauterine system: biological bases of their mechanism of action. *Contraception.* 2007;75(6 Suppl):16-30
3. Sheppard BL. Endometrial morphological changes in IUD users: a review. *Contraception.* 1987; 36(1):1-10
4. Attia AM, Ibrahim MM, Abou-Setta AM. Role of the levonorgestrel intrauterine system in effective contraception. *Patient Prefer Adherence.* 2013;7:777-785
5. American College of Obstetricians and Gynecologists Committee on Practice Bulletins-Gynecology and the Long-Acting Reversible Contraception Work Group. ACOG Practice Bulletin No. 186: Long-acting reversible contraception: implants and intrauterine devices. *Obstet Gynecol.* 2017;130(5):e251-e269
6. American College of Obstetricians and Gynecologists. Facts are important: the start of pregnancy. 2014. https://www.acog.org/-/media/Departments/Government-Relations-and-Outreach/FactsAreImportantPreg.pdf?dmc=1&ts=20180902T1558299894. Accessed September 9, 2018
7. American College of Obstetricians and Gynecologists Committee on Adolescent Health Care. ACOG Committee Opinion No. 392, December 2007. Intrauterine device and adolescents. *Obstet Gynecol.* 2007;110:1493-1495

8. American College of Obstetricians and Gynecologists Committee on Adolescent Health Care and Long-Acting Reversible Contraception Work Group. ACOG Committee Opinion No. 735: adolescents and long-acting reversible contraception: implants and intrauterine devices. *Obstet Gynecol.* 2018;131(5):e130-e139
9. Ott M, Sucato GS; Committee on Adolescence. Contraception for adolescents. *Pediatrics.* 2014;134(4):e1244-e1256
10. Curtis KM, Tepper NK, Jatlaoui TC, et al. U.S. Medical Eligibility Criteria for Contraceptive Use, 2016. *MMWR Recomm Rep.* 2016;65(3):1-103
11. Jatlaoui TC, Riley HEM, Curtis KM. The safety of intrauterine devices among young women: a systematic review. *Contraception.* 2017;95(1):17-39
12. Lohr PA, Lyus R, Prager S. Use of intrauterine devices in nulliparous women. *Contraception.* 2017;95(6):529-537
13. Hoopes AJ, Gilmore K, Cady J, Akers AY, Ahrens KR. A qualitative study of factors that influence contraceptive choice among adolescent school-based health center patients. *J Pediatr Adolesc Gynecol.* 2016;29(3):259-264
14. Melo J, Peters M, Teal S, Guiahi M. Adolescent and young women's contraceptive decision-making processes: Choosing "the best method for her." *J Pediatr Adolesc Gynecol.* 2015;28(4):224-228
15. Marshall C, Kandahari N, Raine-Bennett T. Exploring young women's decisional needs for contraceptive method choice: a qualitative study. *Contraception.* 2018;97(3):243-248
16. Madden T, Mullersman JL, Omvig KJ, Secura GM, Peipert JF. Structured contraceptive counseling provided by the contraceptive CHOICE project. *Contraception.* 2013;88(2):243-249
17. Brown MK, Auerswald C, Eyre SL, Deardorff J, Dehlendorf C. Identifying counseling needs of nulliparous adolescent intrauterine contraceptive users: a qualitative approach. *J Adolesc Health.* 2013;52(3):293-300
18. Hoopes AJ, Gilmore K, Cady J, Akers AY, Ahrens K. A qualitative study of factors that influence contraceptive choice among adolescent school-based health center patients. *J Pediatr Adolesc Gynecol.* 2016;29(3):259-264
19. Potter J, Rubin SE, Sherman P. Fear of intrauterine contraception among adolescents in New York City. *Contraception.* 2014;89(5):446-450
20. Schmidt EO, James A, Curran KM, Peipert JF, Madden T. Adolescent experiences with intrauterine devices: a qualitative study. *J Adolesc Health.* 2015;57(4):381-386
21. Heinemann K, Reed S, Moehner S, Do Minh T. Risk of uterine perforation with levonorgestrel-releasing and copper intrauterine devices in the European Active Surveillance Study on Intrauterine Devices. *Contraception.* 2015;91(4):274-279
22. Hubacher D. Copper intrauterine device use by nulliparous women: review of side effects. *Contraception.* 2007;75(6 Suppl):S8-S11
23. Madden T, McNicholas C, Zhao Q, Secura GM, Eisenberg DL, Peipert JF. Association of age and parity with intrauterine device expulsion. *Obstet Gynecol.* 2014;124(4):718-726
24. Ravi A, Prine L, Waltermaurer E, Miller N, Rubin SE. Intrauterine devices at six months: does patient age matter? Results from an urban family medicine Federally Qualified Health Center (FQHC) network. *J Am Board Fam Med.* 2014;27(6):822-830
25. Aoun J, Dines VA, Stovall DW, Mete M, Nelson CB, Gomez-Lobo V. Effects of age, parity, and device type on complications and discontinuation of intrauterine devices. *Obstet Gynecol.* 2014;123(3):585-592
26. United Nations Development Programme, United Nations Population Fund, World Health Organization, World Bank, Special Programme of Research, Development and Research Training in Human Reproduction. Long-term reversible contraception: twelve years of experience with the TCu380A and TCu220C. *Contraception.* 1997;56(6):341-352
27. Trussell J. Contraceptive failure in the United States. *Contraception.* 2011;83(5):397-404
28. Rowe P, Farley T, Peregoudov A, et al; IUD Research Group of the UNDP/UNFPA/WHO/World Bank Special Programme of Research, Development and Research Training in Human Reproduction. Safety and efficacy of a 52 mg levonorgestrel-medicated intrauterine device: a seven year randomized comparative study with the TCu380A. *Contraception.* 2016;93(6):498-506

29. Workowski K, Bolan G; Centers for Disease Control and Prevention. Sexually transmitted diseases treatment guidelines, 2015. *MMWR Recomm Reports.* 2015;64(3):1-137
30. Weston MRS, Martins SL, Neustadt AB, Gilliam ML. Factors influencing uptake of intrauterine devices among postpartum adolescents: a qualitative study. *Am J Obstet Gynecol.* 2012;206(1): 40.e1-40.e7
31. Fleming KL, Sokoloff A, Raine TR. Attitudes and beliefs about the intrauterine device among teenagers and young women. *Contraception.* 2010;82(2):178-182
32. Kavanaugh ML, Frohwirth L, Jerman J, Popkin R, Ethier K. Long-acting reversible contraception for adolescents and young adults: patient and provider perspectives. *J Pediatr Adolesc Gynecol.* 2013;26(2):86-95
33. Dina B, Peipert LJ, Zhao Q, Peipert JF. Anticipated pain as a predictor of discomfort with intrauterine device placement. *Am J Obstet Gynecol.* 2018;218(2):236.e1-236.e9
34. Bahamondes L, Mansour D, Fiala C, Kaunitz AM, Gemzell-Danielsson K. Practical advice for avoidance of pain associated with insertion of intrauterine contraceptives. *J Fam Plan Reprod Heal Care.* 2014;40(1):54-60
35. Lopez LM, Bernholc A, Zeng Y, et al. Interventions for pain with intrauterine device insertion. *Cochrane Database Syst Rev.* 2015;7:CD007373
36. Rapkin RB, Achilles SL, Schwarz EB, et al. Self-administered lidocaine gel for intrauterine device insertion in nulliparous women: a randomized controlled trial. *Obstet Gynecol.* 2016;128(3): 621-628
37. Akers AY, Steinway C, Sonalkar S, et al. Reducing pain during intrauterine device insertion: a randomized controlled trial in adolescents and young women. *Obstet Gynecol.* 2017;130(4): 795-802
38. Gemzell-Danielsson K, Mansour D, Fiala C, Kaunitz AM, Bahamondes L. Management of pain associated with the insertion of intrauterine contraceptives. *Hum Reprod Update.* 2013;19(4): 419-427
39. Ngo LL, Ward KK, Mody SK. Ketorolac for pain control with intrauterine device placement: a randomized controlled trial. *Obstet Gynecol.* 2015;26(1):29-36
40. Crawford M, Davy S, Book N, Elliott JO, Arora A. Oral ketorolac for pain relief during intrauterine device insertion: a double-blinded randomized controlled trial. *J Obstet Gynaecol Can.* 2017; 39(12):1143-1149
41. Bahamondes MV, Espejo-Arce X, Bahamondes L. Effect of vaginal administration of misoprostol before intrauterine contraceptive insertion following previous insertion failure: a double blind RCT. *Hum Reprod.* 2015;30(8):1861-1866
42. Matthews LR, O'Dwyer L, O'Neill E. Intrauterine device insertion failure after misoprostol administration. *Obstet Gynecol.* 2016;128(5):1084-1091
43. American College of Obstetricians and Gynecologists Committee on Adolescent Health Care. ACOG Committee Opinion No. 448: Menstrual manipulation for adolescents with disabilities. *Obstet Gynecol.* 2009;114(6):1428-1431
44. American College of Obstetricians and Gynecologists' Committee on Gynecologic Practice, Long-Acting Reversible Contraceptive Expert Working Group. ACOG Committee Opinion No. 672: Clinical challenges of long-acting reversible contraceptive methods. 2016;128(3):e69-e77
45. Curtis KM, Jatlaoui TC, Tepper NK, et al. U.S. Selected Practice Recommendations for Contraceptive Use, 2016. *MMWR Recomm Reports.* 2016;65(4):1-66
46. Diedrich JT, Desai S, Zhao Q, Secura G, Madden T, Peipert JF. Association of short-term bleeding and cramping patterns with long-acting reversible contraceptive method satisfaction. *Am J Obstet Gynecol.* 2015;212(1):50.e1-50.e8
47. Hidalgo M, Bahamondes L, Perrotti M, Diaz J, Dantas-Monteiro C, Petta C. Bleeding patterns and clinical performance of the levonorgestrel-releasing intrauterine system (Mirena) up to two years. *Contraception.* 2002;65(2):129-132
48. Mirena Prescribing Information. Bayer Healthcare Pharmaceuticals. http://labeling.bayerhealthcare.com/html/products/pi/Mirena_PI.pdf. Accessed September 26, 2016

49. Skyla Prescribing Information. Bayer Healthcare Pharmaceuticals. http://labeling.bayerhealthcare.com/html/products/pi/Skyla_PI.pdf. Accessed September 26, 2016
50. Godfrey EM, Folger SG, Jeng G, Jamieson DJ, Curtis KM. Treatment of bleeding irregularities in women with copper-containing IUDs: a systematic review. *Contraception*. 2013;87(5):549-566
51. Allen R, Villavicencio J. Unscheduled bleeding and contraceptive choice: increasing satisfaction and continuation rates. *Open Access J Contracept*. 2016;7:43-52
52. Stanwood NL, Bradley KA. Young pregnant women's knowledge of modern intrauterine devices. *Obstet Gynecol*. 2006;108(6):1417-1422
53. Whitaker AK, Johnson LM, Harwood B, Chiappetta L, Creinin MD, Gold MA. Adolescent and young adult women's knowledge of and attitudes toward the intrauterine device. *Contraception*. 2008;78(3):211-217
54. Barrett M, Soon R, Whitaker AK, Takekawa S, Kaneshiro B. Awareness and knowledge of the intrauterine device in adolescents. *J Pediatr Adolesc Gynecol*. 2012;25(1):39-42
55. Spies EL, Askelson NM, Gelman E, Losch M. Young women's knowledge, attitudes, and behaviors related to long-acting reversible contraceptives. *Womens Health Issues*. 2010;20(6):394-399
56. Hladky KJ, Allsworth JE, Madden T, Secura GM, Peipert JF. Women's knowledge about intrauterine contraception. *Obstet Gynecol*. 2011;117(1):48-54
57. Finer LB, Jerman J, Kavanaugh ML. Changes in use of long-acting contraceptive methods in the United States, 2007–2009. *Fertil Steril*. 2012;98(4):893–897
58. Abma JC, Martinez G. Sexual activity and contraceptive use among teenagers in the United States, 2011–2015. *Natl Health Stat Rep*. 2017;104:1-23
59. Romero L, Pazol K, Warner L, et al. Vital signs: trends in use of long-acting reversible contraception among teens aged 15–19 years seeking contraceptive services—United States, 2005–2013. *MMWR Morb Mortality Wkly Rep*. 2015;64(13):363-369
60. Cohen R, Sheeder J, Kane M, Teal SB. Factors associated with contraceptive method choice and initiation in adolescents and young women. *J Adolesc*. 2017;61:454-460
61. Mestad R, Secura G, Allsworth JE, Madden T, Zhao Q, Peipert JF. Acceptance of long-acting reversible contraceptive methods by adolescent participants in the Contraceptive CHOICE Project. *Contraception*. 2011;84(5):493-498
62. Hoopes AJ, Teal SB, Akers AY, Sheeder J. Low acceptability of certain contraceptive methods among young women. *J Pediatr Adolesc Gynecol*. 2018;31(3):274-280
63. Antonishak J, Kaye K, Swaider L. Impact of an online birth control support network on unintended pregnancy. *Soc Mar Q*. 2015;21(1):23-36
64. Secura GM, Allsworth JE, Madden T, Mullersman JL, Peipert JF. The Contraceptive CHOICE Project: reducing barriers to long-acting reversible contraception. *Am J Obstet Gynecol*. 2010;203(2):115.e1-115.e7
65. Winner B, Peipert JF, Zhao Q, et al. Effectiveness of long-acting reversible contraception. *N Engl J Med*. 2012;366(21):1998-2007
66. Ricketts S, Klingler G, Schwalberg R. Game change in Colorado: widespread use of long-acting reversible contraceptives and rapid decline in births among young, low-income women. *Perspect Sex Reprod Health*. 2014;46(3):125-132
67. Rubin SE, Davis K, McKee MD. New York City physicians' views of providing long-acting reversible contraception to adolescents. *Ann Fam Med*. 2013;11(2):130-136
68. Wilson SF, Strohsnitter W, Baecher-Lind L. Practices and perceptions among pediatricians regarding adolescent contraception with emphasis on intrauterine contraception. *J Pediatr Adolesc Gynecol*. 2013;26(5):281-284
69. Swanson KJ, Gossett DR, Fournier M. Pediatricians' beliefs and prescribing patterns of adolescent contraception: a provider survey. *J Pediatr Adolesc Gynecol*. 2013;26(6):340-345
70. Kohn JE, Hacker JG, Rousselle MA, Gold M. Knowledge and likelihood to recommend intrauterine devices for adolescents among school-based health center providers. *J Adolesc Heal*. 2012;51(4):319-324
71. Pritt NM, Norris AH, Berlan ED. Barriers and facilitators to adolescents' use of long-acting reversible contraceptives. *J Pediatr Adolesc Gynecol*. 2017;30(1):18-22

72. Greenberg KB, Makino KK, Coles MS. Factors associated with provision of long-acting reversible contraception among adolescent health care providers. *J Adolesc Health*. 2013;52(3):372-374
73. Potter J, Koyama A, Coles MS. Addressing the challenges of clinician training for long-acting reversible contraception. *JAMA Pediatr*. 2015;169(2):103-104
74. Upstream USA. https://www.upstream.org/approach/. Accessed November 18, 2018
75. Welti K, Manlove J. Unintended pregnancy in Delaware: estimating change after the first two years of an intervention to increase contraceptive access. Child Trends. March 14, 2018. https://www.childtrends.org/publications/unintended-pregnancy-delaware-estimating-change-first-two-years-intervention-increase-contraceptive-access. Accessed November 18, 2018
76. Gilmore K, Hoopes AJ, Cady J, Amies Oelschlager A-M, Prager S, Vander Stoep A. Providing long-acting reversible contraception services in Seattle school-based health centers: Key themes for facilitating implementation. *J Adolesc Health*. 2015;56(6):658-665
77. Hoopes AJ, Sucato GS, Diekema DS. Involving parents in pediatric patients' decisions about long-acting reversible contraception. *JAMA Pediatr*. 2016;170(5):409-410
78. Grunloh DS, Casner T, Secura GM, Peipert JF, Madden T. Characteristics associated with discontinuation of long-acting reversible contraception within the first 6 months of use. *Obstet Gynecol*. 2013;122(6):1214-1221
79. Ross L; SisterSong Women of Color Reproductive Health Collective. Understanding Reproductive Justice. 2006. https://d3n8a8pro7vhmx.cloudfront.net/rrfp/pages/33/attachments/original/1456425809/Understanding_RJ_Sistersong.pdf?1456425809. Accessed September 9, 2018
80. Horton LG, Folger SG, Berry-Bibee E, Jatlaoui TC, Tepper NK, Curtis KM. Research gaps from evidence-based contraception guidance: the US Medical Eligibility Criteria for Contraceptive Use, 2016 and the US Selected Practice Recommendations for Contraceptive Use, 2016. *Contraception*. 2016;94(6):582-589

Adolesc Med 030 (2019) 118–133

A "Call To Arms": Using the Contraceptive Implant to Reduce Unplanned Adolescent Pregnancy

Kathryn Gannon-Loew, MD, MS[a]; Casey Cottrill, MD, MPH[b]; Elise Berlan, MD, MPH[c*]

[a]Adolescent Medicine Fellow, Nationwide Children's Hospital, Columbus, Ohio; [b]Assistant Professor of Pediatrics, The Ohio State University College of Medicine, Division of Adolescent Medicine, Nationwide Children's Hospital, Columbus, Ohio; [c]Associate Professor of Pediatrics, The Ohio State University College of Medicine, Division of Adolescent Medicine, Nationwide Children's Hospital, Columbus Ohio

LEARNING OBJECTIVES

After reviewing this article, the reader should be able to:

1. Describe the effectiveness and indications for use of the etonogestrel implant
2. Enumerate the side effects and management of the etonogestrel implant
3. Outline the steps for insertion of the etonogestrel implant
4. List complications of the etonogestrel implant

INTRODUCTION

The etonogestrel (ENG) implant Nexplanon is a long-acting reversible contraceptive that provides effective contraception for 3 years. Given its convenience, Nexplanon is a desirable choice for contraception for many adolescents and is recommended as first-line contraceptive options for adolescents.[1] It is important for physicians and other clinicians who care for adolescents to be comfortable counseling patients about this option. This article will review background information on Nexplanon, its use in adolescents, indications and contraindications, side effects, and complications. Management options for irregular menstrual bleeding, the most common side effect associated with Nexplanon, are discussed.

*Corresponding author
E-mail address: Elise.Berlan@nationwidechildrens.org

 ISSN 1934-4287

BACKGROUND

The Implant

The ENG implant, currently available in the United States as Nexplanon (Merck, Whitehouse Station, NJ), replaced Implanon when it was introduced in 2011. Nexplanon is a cylindrical rod (4 cm long × 2 mm in diameter) placed subdermally in the upper arm. The ENG is embedded in a core of ethylene vinyl acetate that allows for slow release of the hormone. In contrast to Implanon, Nexplanon contains barium sulfate, making the implant radiopaque. This allows the device to be located by plain film, ultrasound, computed tomography, and magnetic resonance imaging if it cannot be palpated. Additionally, Nexplanon comes preloaded in a disposable applicator, which prevents deep insertion and maintains the device in the sterile applicator until insertion is completed.

Nexplanon contains 68 mg of ENG, the active metabolite of desogestrel, a third-generation progestin (Figure 1). After insertion, levels of ENG rise rapidly, reaching a mean ENG concentration of 265.9 pg/mL at 8 hours and maximize concentration between days 1 and 13 after insertion. Mean concentration at 1 year is 196 pg/mL.[2] The primary mechanism of action is inhibition of ovulation,[3] with ENG levels greater than 90 pg/mL shown to prevent ovulation.[4] ENG also thickens cervical mucus[3,5] and affects the endometrium, although the mechanism is not fully understood.[6,7] The implant is effective 24 to 48 hours after insertion,[5] and ovulation resumes for many users within 10 days to 2 weeks after removal.[2] Concentrations of ENG remain sufficient to inhibit ovulation throughout its period of use.[8]

Effectiveness

The ENG implant is more than 99% effective at preventing pregnancy and is approved by the US Food and Drug Administration for 3 years of use. Implanon and Nexplanon are biologically equivalent, and studies of effectiveness were primarily conducted on Implanon. In 11 international clinical trials on Implanon, of the 923 women included in the analysis of efficacy, no pregnancies occurred while the implant was in place.[9] Six pregnancies occurred within 14 days after

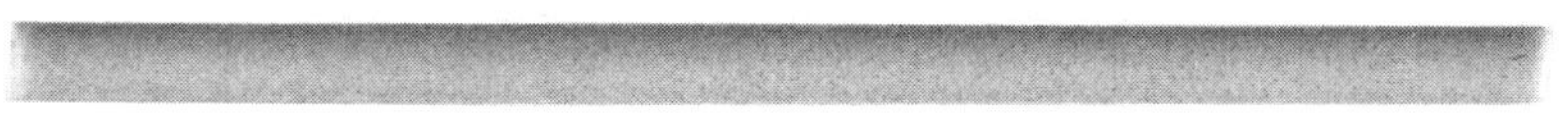

Fig 1. Photograph of Nexplanon.

the implant was removed. Including those 6 pregnancies, the cumulative Pearl index (expected number of pregnancies per 100 woman-years of exposure) for subjects younger than 35 years was 0.38. In a postmarketing analysis in Australia 3 years after the availability of Implanon, the failure rate was estimated to be 1 in 1000 cases.[10] Of 127 reported cases of unintended pregnancy with Implanon, the most common reason was failure to insert the implant (n = 84). Changes in the Nexplanon applicator have helped prevent this complication.

Nexplanon seems to be effective beyond 3 years. In a prospective cohort study of 291 ENG users, no pregnancies were documented during the additional 2 year postexpiration period.[11] Similarly, in a study of 204 women with the ENG implant, no pregnancies were reported among participants using the implant for 5 years.[12]

Uptake and Continuation

The ENG implant is an appealing option for contraception for many women. The Contraceptive CHOICE Project was a prospective cohort of more than 9000 women aged 14 to 45 years seeking a new contraceptive method who were offered their choice of contraception free of charge. Seventeen percent of all participants in the Contraceptive CHOICE Project chose the ENG implant.[13] Specifically, among 14- to 17-year-olds, 43% chose the implant and among 18- to 20-year-olds 17% chose the implant.[14] In a retrospective cohort study examining uptake of ENG implants versus intrauterine devices over 4 years, among 249 females younger than 20 years, uptake of the implant was significantly greater than that of the intrauterine device (IUD) (54.6% vs 45.4%).[15]

Studies have also demonstrated high rates of continuation among users of the ENG implant. In the Contraceptive CHOICE Project, continuation of the ENG implant was 82% at year 1, 69% at year 2, and 56% at year 3. This was higher compared to continuation of non-LARC methods overall.[16] A secondary analysis of this study found that among nulliparous women 14 to 19 years old (n = 614), the continuation rate was 83% at 12 months and 65% at 24 months.[17] Other studies of ENG implant use in adolescents and young adults have demonstrated high rates of continuation. A retrospective chart review of 94 adolescents with ENG implants found a continuation rate of 78% at 12 months, 50% at 24 months, and 40% at 32 months.[18] A retrospective chart review of 750 females aged 12 to 22 years found that 10.3% of patients had the device removed before 12 months of use, and problematic bleeding was the most common reason for early removal.[19] In this study, older age at time of insertion, history of pregnancy, and having at least 1 medical visit for implant concerns were predictive of discontinuing the implant. A systematic review evaluating 12-month continuation of LARCs in adolescents and young adults found an overall ENG implant continuation rate of 84%.[20]

Studies have also assessed continuation in special populations of adolescents. In a secondary analysis of the Contraceptive CHOICE Project, among 249 parous adolescents aged 14 to 19 years, continuation of the ENG implant was 92% at 12 months and 72% at 24 months.[17] In a prospective cohort study, 171 postpartum 13- to 24-year-olds who chose the subdermal implant were compared to a control group of 225 postpartum subjects who chose any other method of contraception.[21] Continuation of the implant was 97% at 6 months and 86% at 12 months. In another study of postpartum adolescents, ENG implant users were more likely to continue using their method compared to users of oral contraceptives or depot medroxyprogesterone acetate (DMPA).[22]

However, when ENG implants are compared to IUDs, implants are more likely to be discontinued. A randomized, open-label, phase 3 study compared the levonorgestrel intrauterine system (LNG-IUS) to the ENG implant in women aged 18 to 35 years and found the 12-month discontinuation rate was significantly higher in the ENG implant group (26.8%) compared to the LNG-IUS group (19.6%).[23] A greater proportion of women in the ENG implant group discontinued use because of increased bleeding (11.3% vs 3.2%).[23] Another study comparing the LNG-IUS to the ENG implant found similar results; women with implants were more likely to discontinue early than women with LNG-IUS (47% vs 27%).[24] Specifically in adolescents, in a study of health insurance claims (2007-2011), among 2388 youth aged 15 to 19 years, 12.4% had the implant removed within 1 year; this was not significantly different from removal of LNG-IUS.[25] However, among 20- to 24-year-olds, removal of the ENG implant was significantly higher than removal of LNG-IUS.

INDICATIONS AND CONTRAINDICATIONS

Medical Eligibility Criteria

According to the Centers for Disease Control and Prevention (CDC) 2016 U.S. Medical Eligibility Criteria for Contraceptive Use (US MEC), there are no restrictions on use of the ENG implant based on age.[26] The implant can safely be inserted immediately postpartum and postabortion.[27] In breastfeeding women, initiation of ENG implant is US MEC category 1 (there is no restriction) or 2 (advantages generally outweigh the theoretical proven risks), depending on the timing of insertion (Table 1). Placement of the implant is classified as US MEC category 2 in breastfeeding women less than 30 days postpartum because of theoretical concerns about milk production; however, small studies have found no difference in milk production between those who received the implant immediately postpartum compared to those with no contraception or delayed insertion.[28,29]

Table 1
Selected U.S. Medical Eligibility Criteria and contraceptive implant

MEC category 1	MEC category 2	MEC category 3	MEC category 4
• Postpartum (non-breastfeeding) • Postpartum ≥30 days (breastfeeding)	• Postpartum <30 days (breastfeeding)	• Breast cancer: past and no evidence of current disease for 5 years • Severe (compensated) cirrhosis • Hepatocellular adenoma • Malignant liver tumor • Systemic lupus erythematosus in which antiphospholipid antibodies are present or unknown • Unexplained vaginal bleeding (suspicious for serious condition) • Continuation in the setting of ischemic heart disease and stroke	• Current breast cancer

MEC, U.S. Medical Eligibility Criteria for Contraceptive Use.
Derived from Curtis K, Tepper N, Jatlaoui T, et al. U.S. Medical Eligibility Criteria for Contraceptive Use, 2016. *MMWR Recomm Rep.* 2016;65(3):1-103

There are a limited number of circumstances for which use of the implant is not recommended. The implant is US MEC category 3 (theoretical or proven risks usually outweigh the advantages) if a woman has a history of breast cancer and category 4 (unacceptable health risk) for those with current breast cancer. It is US MEC category 3 for use in women with severe cirrhosis, hepatocellular adenoma and malignant liver tumors, systemic lupus erythematosus in which antiphospholipid antibodies are present or unknown, and unexplained vaginal bleeding (suspicious for serious condition) before an evaluation. In addition, it is US MEC category 3 for continuation in the setting of ischemic heart disease and stroke (for additional information about US MEC, see the article on adolescent pregnancy prevention and application of CDC evidence-based contraception guidance by Zapata et al in this issue of AM:STARs).

Dysmenorrhea

In addition to its role as a contraceptive, Nexplanon has non-contraceptive benefits, particularly for dysmenorrhea. In data from 11 clinical trials, 77% of patients with dysmenorrhea before placement had complete resolution.[30] In a study of 315 women, among those with dysmenorrhea at baseline, 81% had improvement in symptoms.[31] When compared to DMPA, 68% of women with ENG implant had improvement of dysmenorrhea compared to 53% of women using DMPA.[32]

Use in Select Populations: Overweight and Obesity

Studies have demonstrated the effectiveness of ENG implant in women who are overweight and obese. The Contraceptive CHOICE Project found that the 3-year cumulative failure rates for women with the ENG implant did not vary by body mass index.[33] A cross-sectional study of females aged 18 to 44 years found comparable levels of ENG across women of normal weight, women who were overweight, and women who were obese.[34]

INSERTION AND REMOVAL

The implant is easy to insert and remove by trained providers. Health care professionals, including physicians, advance practice nurses, and physician assistants, are required to complete a 2-hour hands-on training session to become eligible to place implants.

The ENG implant may be inserted at any time during the menstrual cycle, as long as pregnancy can be reasonably excluded.[35] If the implant is inserted within 5 days of the start of menstrual bleeding, a backup contraceptive is not needed. If it is inserted more than 5 days from the start of the menstrual cycle, it is possible that ovulation has already occurred, and it is recommended that the woman abstain or use a barrier method for 7 days after insertion. If the clinician is uncertain whether the woman is pregnant, the benefits of starting the implant likely outweigh the risk, and the clinician can consider placing the implant at any time, with a follow-up pregnancy test in 2 to 4 weeks.[35]

The Nexplanon applicator was designed to allow insertion with 1 hand, prevent deep insertion, and keep the implant in place within the applicator before insertion.[27] The device should be inserted on the medial surface of the non-dominant arm, 8 to 10 cm proximal to the medical epicondyle of the humerus, over the triceps muscle, and placed just below the skin to avoid the neurovascular bundle.[36] After insertion, the device should be palpated by the patient and clinician to ensure placement. The patient should be advised to return at any time to discuss adverse effects, if she is considering an alternative method of contraception, and when it is time for removal.

Complications are uncommon at the time of implant insertion (1.0%) and removal (1.7%).[9] In a study of more than 20,000 Implanon insertions reported as part of a voluntary active monitoring program, insertion-related events occurred in 1% of patients, and removal-related events occurred in 6.3%.[37] As with any procedure, the risks and potential complications should be discussed before placement. Insertion complications include pain, bleeding, hematoma, infection, scarring, deep or improper insertion, and unrecognized non-insertion. Although modifications were made to the applicator to prevent deep insertions, case reports demonstrate that this event can still occur.[38]

The implant is removed by making a small incision over its distal end. The rod may be covered by a fibrous capsule that must be released. If desired, a new implant can be inserted through the same incision used for removal if it is properly positioned. Removal complications include breakage of the implant or inability to palpate the implant, requiring imaging before removal.[27] If at any time during its use the implant is not palpated, pregnancy should be excluded and a backup method of contraception or emergency contraception used until the presence of the implant is confirmed and the implant is removed.

SIDE EFFECTS OF THE IMPLANT

Abnormal Menstrual Bleeding

Prevalence of Bleeding

Abnormal menstrual bleeding is reported as the most frequent side effect associated with the ENG implant. Meta-analysis data from 11 clinical trials demonstrated abnormal menstrual bleeding was common and included amenorrhea (22.2%), infrequent bleeding (33.6%), frequent bleeding (6.7%), and prolonged bleeding (17.7%); approximately 11% of women discontinued the implant because of irregular bleeding.[30] In the Contraceptive CHOICE Project, of the

1184 women using the ENG implant, at 3 months 42% reported decreased bleeding frequency and 35% reported increased bleeding, and at 6 months 48% reported decreased bleeding frequency and 21% reported increased bleeding.[16] A retrospective study of health insurance claims compared women aged 15 to 44 years with LNG-IUS (n = 79,920) versus ENG implants (n = 7374) from 2007 to 2012. Users of ENG across all age groups were more likely to experience irregular menstrual bleeding within 1 year of insertion compared to LNG-IUS users.[25]

Abnormal bleeding may lead to more frequent visits to a health care professional or early discontinuation. A retrospective chart review of 155 women with ENG implants found that 27% saw a health care professional for bleeding concerns.[32] In a study comparing LNG-IUS to ENG implants, among the 147 implant users, dissatisfaction with bleeding pattern was the most common reason for discontinuation.[24] In a study of semistructured interviews with 18 women, bleeding was the main reason that prompted implant removal.[39] In adolescents specifically, a retrospective chart review of 94 adolescents aged 13 to 22 years with an ENG implant found that 48% experienced nuisance bleeding, and 63% of those patients received medication management for the bleeding; early implant removal because of bleeding occurred in 18%.[18]

Anticipatory Counseling

Given the frequency of abnormal bleeding, adequate anticipatory counseling before insertion is important. Patients should be counseled that unpredictable light bleeding or spotting is common and that heavy or frequent bleeding or no bleeding may also occur.

Vaginal bleeding during the first 3 months after insertion may predict the pattern of bleeding. Women with favorable bleeding during that time tend to continue with that same pattern, but at least 50% of women with initial negative bleeding will have an improvement over time.[30,31,40]

Management of Unscheduled Bleeding Secondary to Implant

Before discussing treatment options, the clinician should obtain a detailed history of the bleeding pattern and rule out other causes of bleeding, such as ectopic pregnancy and sexually transmitted infections as indicated. Because the exact etiology of bleeding with Nexplanon is unknown, treatment options are aimed at different mechanisms that may be contributing to the bleeding pattern[41]; however, a discussion of all aspects of irregular bleeding secondary to an implant is beyond the scope of this article.

Nonsteroidal anti-inflammatory drugs (NSAIDs) act by inhibiting cyclooxygenase, thereby decreasing prostaglandins that could be contributing to the bleeding. In a randomized controlled trial, ENG implant users receiving mefenamic acid had fewer bleeding episodes over 4 weeks compared to placebo (10.5 vs 16.8 days; $P < .05$).[42] A retrospective cohort study evaluated reassurance only versus reassurance and ibuprofen and found that the ENG implant discontinuation rate did not differ between the 2 groups.[43] According to U.S. Selected Practice Recommendations for Contraceptive Use, a 5- to 7-day course of NSAIDs can be considered for treatment of bothersome bleeding.[35]

Estrogen, including combined oral contraceptives (COCs), may decrease bleeding by stabilizing the endometrial lining. In a double-blind, randomized controlled trial of 26 women reporting bothersome bleeding, participants were randomized to COC or placebo; 92% of COC users compared to 42% of placebo users reported significant improvement in bleeding at 4 weeks ($P = .03$).[44] In a randomized trial of 32 women with bothersome bleeding, women randomized to 14 days of COC were more likely to have temporary interruption of bleeding compared to placebo.[45] However, bleeding resumed in 86% of patients within 10 days of stopping treatment.[45]

Doxycycline, another management option, works by inhibiting matrix metalloproteinase activity, which may play a role in endometrial tissue remodeling and potentially contribute to unscheduled bleeding. In a randomized controlled trial of ENG implant users, 45 participants receiving doxycycline demonstrated faster time to bleeding cessation compared to participants receiving placebo (4.8 days vs 7.5 days).[46] A follow-up study failed to support these findings.[47] A retrospective cohort study of ENG implant users found that patients receiving doxycycline had significantly lower discontinuation rates than patients receiving reassurance alone ($P = .005$).[43] A suggested dose is 100 mg twice daily for 5 days.

Tranexamic acid (TXA) may be another therapeutic option for treatment of breakthrough bleeding. TXA is an antifibrinolytic that decreases clot breakdown and thus bleeding, and it has been shown to be effective for treatment of unscheduled bleeding with DMPA use. Among implant users, TXA resulted in a greater proportion of participants experiencing bleeding cessation during the first week, but the difference did not persist at 4 weeks.[48] The dosage for TXA can be extrapolated from that used for abnormal uterine bleeding and is given at 1300 mg 3 times daily by mouth for 5 days.[41]

Mifepristone is an antiprogestin that upregulates estrogen receptors in the endometrium, potentially stabilizing the endometrium. In a randomized controlled trial of ENG implant users with bleeding, the use of mifepristone demonstrated no improvement in time to bleeding cessation compared to placebo (5.9 days vs 7.5 days).[46] However, the use of mifepristone for 1 day followed by estradiol for 4 days resulted in a significant decrease in time to bleeding cessation compared to placebo (4.3 days vs 7.5 days).[46] In a follow-up study, when mifepristone was followed by doxycycline for 5 days, there was a significant decrease in time to bleeding cessation compared to placebo (4.4 days vs 6.4 days).[47] The availability of mifepristone may limit its use.

Finally, tamoxifen is a selective estrogen receptor modulator that may antagonize the angiogenic effect of estrogen.[41] Two small randomized controlled trials of tamoxifen compared to placebo demonstrated improvement in bleeding.[49,50] The dose of tamoxifen was 10 mg twice daily for 7 days.[50]

Overall, there are several options for a clinician to consider when patients present with bothersome bleeding secondary to Nexplanon. According to U.S. Selected Practice Recommendations for Contraceptive Use, NSAIDs or hormonal treatment with low-dose COC or estrogen should be given for short-term treatment of bothersome bleeding associated with the ENG implant.[35]

Other Side Effects of the Implant

Aside from unscheduled bleeding, other reported side effects include headache (15.5%), weight gain (12.0%), acne (11.8%), breast pain (10.2%), emotional lability (5.8%), and abdominal pain (5.2%).[9] However, findings are mixed regarding the effect on the ENG implant on acne. A non-comparative multicenter controlled study of more than 600 women using the ENG implant found that acne developed or worsened in 12.6% and improved in 12.8% of participants.[3] In a study of 315 women using the ENG implant, 16% reported decreased acne, 70% reported no change, and 14% reported an increase in acne.[31] Other studies have demonstrated that between 10% and 14% of users experience worsening acne, but less than 2% discontinue use for this reason.[9,31]

Additional studies have evaluated the effect of the ENG implant on weight and metabolic changes. In an analysis of 11 international clinical trials on Implanon, 12% reported weight gain and 2.3% discontinued because of this weight increase.[9] Similar results were found in a multicenter clinical trial of 330 women with Implanon, with about 12% of participants reporting weight increase.[31] In a study of 44 adolescents with the ENG implant, in the first year after placement no changes in mean body weight, body mass index, or blood pressure were reported.[51] In a 3-year prospective cohort study of 213 females aged 22 to 32 years, weight increased on average 3 kg (P = .16) and body mass index increased 1 kg/m^2 (P = .05).[52] Participants experienced no significant change in blood pressure; fasting blood glucose levels increased but remained within a normal range. There was a significant reduction in high-density lipoprotein and a trend toward reductions in triglycerides and low-density lipoprotein. Other studies have found similar effects on cholesterol, with implant users experiencing a decrease in total cholesterol, low-density lipoprotein, high-density lipoprotein, and triglycerides.[53,54]

A small body of evidence on the effect of the ENG implant on bone health has been reported. A prospective study comparing ENG implant users to non-hormonal IUD users found no statistically difference in bone mineral density between the 2 groups.[55] A randomized controlled trial in 111 women aged 19 to

43 years comparing ENG implant versus levonorgestrel implant found bone mineral density was significantly decreased in both groups at the midshaft of the ulna at 18 months, although the decrease was not outside 1 standard deviation.[56] There was no significant difference at the distal radius. The clinical significance of these changes is unclear.

Side effects of the ENG implant may result in visits to a health care professional or early removal of the implant. In a retrospective study of 155 implant users, 64 saw a health care professional for implant-related concerns: the majority were related to bleeding, followed by weight gain, mood changes, and headaches.[32] In semistructured interviews of 18 women, reasons for early removal in addition to bleeding included mood swings, weight gain, and cosmetic side effects such as scarring and acne.[39]

Drug Interactions

Drugs that induce the liver cytochrome p450 system may reduce serum concentrations of concomitantly used ethinyl estradiol and progestins and therefore may reduce their contraceptive efficacy. This area is not well investigated. A few studies have evaluated the interaction between the ENG implant and specific medications. In a single study, in 95% of patients taking efavirenz as antiretroviral therapy for human immunodeficiency virus, ENG plasma concentration levels were below the threshold thought to suppress ovulation (90 pg/mL) at 24 weeks.[57] There are 2 reported cases on unintended pregnancy in patients with the ENG implant taking efavirenz.[58] In a study of carbamazepine use in 10 ENG implant users, median ENG concentrations decreased significantly after carbamazepine administration; in 8 of 10 participants, ENG concentration was below the level for ovulatory suppression.[59] Physicians should consider potential medication interactions when counseling patients about the implant and refer to up-to-date clinical guidance, when available.

COMPLICATIONS

Several studies and numerous case reports have investigated complications associated with Implanon and Nexplanon. Rare but serious complications include broken implants, migration, and implant site reactions. In a survey of physicians evaluating fracture rates with different types of hormonal implants, 54 fractures were reported, 70% with Nexplanon. The mechanisms of fracture included patient manipulation, unintentional trauma, interpersonal violence, lifting/carrying, and fracture on removal.[60] Complications with migration to a distant site have also been reported. A study using the US Food and Drug Administration Adverse Event Reporting System database identified 38 cases of ENG implant migration to locations such as the lung and pulmonary artery, chest wall, vasculature other than the lung/pulmonary artery, and extravascular locations including the axilla, clavicle, and shoulder.[61] Several case reports describe insertion into the venous system resulting in embolism to the pulmonary artery.[62-66] Insertion above or below rather than in the sulcus between the biceps and triceps may prevent this rare complication. Other case reports describe migration to the axilla.[67,68] Multiple imaging techniques including radiography, ultrasound, and computed tomography can be helpful in localizing the implant if it is not palpable. In addition, an ENG level can be used to determine whether the implant is present in the body. Other complications include median nerve injury after implant removal[69] and implant site reactions.[70,71]

CONCLUSION

Overall, Nexplanon is a highly effective contraceptive method that is easy to place and remove. It is desirable option for many adolescents as maintenance does not require any additional actions from the user. It is important for health care professionals to provide adequate anticipatory counseling about potential side effects, including irregular bleeding, which may result in dissatisfaction or early discontinuation of the implant.

QUESTIONS

1. A 20-year-old female is in your office to discuss contraception options. She is finishing college next year and plans to get married to her long-term boyfriend at that time. She is anticipating trying to get pregnant shortly after getting married. She has a history of deep vein thrombosis in her left leg 2 years ago. She tells you that she desires the most effective contraception available until she is ready to get pregnant because she wants to finish college without becoming pregnant. Which of the following is the best choice for contraception for this patient?
   A. Etonogestrel implant
   B. Progestin-only pill
   C. Latex condoms
   D. Vaginal ring
2. A 14-year-old female with an etonogestrel implant in place is concerned about irregular bleeding. The implant was placed 1 year ago, and since then she experienced 2 to 3 days of moderate bleeding every 2 to 3 weeks. Her point-of-care hemoglobin test result is normal. She denies any sexual activity within the last year, and her sexually transmitted infection test result is negative from 6 months ago. Which of the following is the first-line medication choice to help this patient with her irregular bleeding?
   A. Tamoxifen 20 mg once daily by mouth for 7 days
   B. Tranexamic acid 1300 mg 3 times per day by mouth for 5 days
   C. Doxycycline 100 mg twice daily by mouth for 5 days
   D. Naproxen 500 mg twice daily for 5 days

3. An 18-year-old female comes to your office for follow-up after being diagnosed with pelvic inflammatory disease 2 days ago. She has been adhering to her antibiotic regimen without difficulty. She has a history of migraine with aura. She is sexually active with 1 male partner and tells you she also is desiring contraception today. Which of the following is true of the most effective contraceptive option for this patient?
   A. Primary mechanism of action is cervical mucus thickening.
   B. Contraceptive effectiveness is achieved only after 14 days of use.
   C. After discontinuation, ovulation resumes within 10 to 14 days.
   D. Contraindicated for use when breastfeeding.

(See page 202 for answers.)

References

1. American Academy of Pediatrics Committee on Adolescence. Policy statement. Contraception for adolescents. *Pediatrics.* 2014;134(4):e1244-e1256
2. Makarainen L, Van Beek A, Tuomivaara L, Asplund B, Coelingh Bennink H. Ovarian function during the use of a single contraceptive implant: Implanon compared with Norplant. *Fertil Steril.* 1998;69:714-721
3. Croxatto H. Mechanisms that explain the contraceptive action of progestin implants for women. *Contraception.* 2002;65:21-27
4. Diaz A, Pavez M, Moo-Young A, Bardin C, Croxatto H. Clinical trial with 3-keto-desogestrel subdermal implants. *Contraception.* 1991;44(4):393-408
5. Davies G, Feng L, Newton J, Van Beek A, Coelingh-Bennink H. Release characteristics, ovarian activity and menstrual bleeding pattern with a single contraceptive implant releasing 3-ketodesogestrel. *Contraception.* 1993;47:251-261
6. Varma R, Mascarenhas L. Endometrial effects of the etonogestrel (Implanon) contraceptive implant. *Curr Opin Obstet Gynecol.* 2001;13:335-341
7. Lortlar N, Kilic S, Peker T, et al. The long-term effects of progesterone-only contraceptives on endometrium and ovary in rats. *Arch Gynecol Obstet.* 2010;281:1051-1059
8. Bennink H. The pharmacokinetics and pharmacodynamics of Implanon, a single rod etonorgestrel contraceptive implant. *Eur J Contracept Reprod Health Care.* 2000;5(Suppl 2):12-20
9. Darney P, Patel A, Rosen K, Shapiro L, Kaunitz A. Safety and efficacy of a single-rod etonogestrel implant (Implanon): results from 11 international clinical trials. *Fertil Steril.* 2009;91:1646-1653
10. Harrison-Woolrych M, Hill R. Unintended pregnancies with the etonogestrel implant (Implanon): a case series from post-marketing experience in Australia. *Contraception.* 2005;71:306-308
11. McNicholas C, Swor E, Wan L, Peipert J. Prolonged use of the etonogestrel implant and levonorgestrel intrauterine device: 2 years beyond Food and Drug Administration-approved duration. *Am J Obstet Gynecol.* 2017;216(6):586.e1-586.e6
12. Ali M, Akin A, Bahamondes L, et al. Extended use up to 5 years of the etonogestrel-releasing subdermal contraceptive implant: comparison to levonorgestrel-releasing subdermal implant. WHO study group on subdermal contraceptive implants for women. *Hum Reprod.* 2016;31: 2491-2498
13. Peipert J, Madden T, Allsworth J, Secura G. Preventing unintended pregnancies by providing no-cost contraception. *Obstet Gynecol.* 2012;120:1291-1297
14. Mestad R, Secura G, Allsworth JE, Madden T, Zhao Q, Peipert JF. Acceptance of long-acting reversible contraceptive methods by adolescent participants in the Contraceptive CHOICE Project. *Contraception.* 2011;84:493-498
15. Howard DL, Ford A, Ceballos S, Volker KW. Temporal trends in the uptake and continuation of the Etonogestrel implant in a large private practice setting. *JWomens Health (Larchmt).* 2018; 27(2):191-195

16. Deidrich J, Zhao Q, Madden T, Secura G, Peipert J. Three-year continuation of reversible contraception. *Am J Obstet Gynecol.* 2015;213(5):662.e1-662.e8
17. Abraham M, Zhao Q, Peipert JF. Young age, nulliparity, and continuation of long-acting reversible contraceptive methods. *Obstet Gynecol.* 2015;126(4):823-829
18. Obijuru L, Bumpus S, Auinger P, Baldwin CD. Etonogestrel implants in adolescents: experience, satisfaction, and continuation. *J Adolesc Health.* 2016;58:284-289
19. Berlan E, Mizraji K, Bonny A. Twelve-month discontinuation of etonogestrel implant in an outpatient pediatric setting. *Contraception.* 2016;94:81-86
20. Diedrich JT, Klein DA, Peipert JF. Long-acting reversible contraception in adolescents: a systematic review and meta-analysis. *Am J Obstet Gynecol.* 2017;216(4):364.e1-364.e12
21. Tocce K, Sheeder J, Teal S. Rapid repeat pregnancy in adolescents: do immediate postpartum contraceptive implants make a difference? *Am J Obstet Gynecol.* 2012;206(6):481.e1-481.e7
22. Lewis L, Doherty D, Hickey M, Skinner S. Implanon as a contraceptive choice for teenage mothers: a comparison of contraceptive choices, acceptability and repeat pregnancy. *Contraception.* 2010;81:421-426
23. Apter D, Briggs P, Tuppurainen M, et al. A 12-month multicenter, randomized study comparing the levonorgestrel intrauterine system with the etonogestrel subdermal implant. *Fertil Steril.* 2016;106(1):151-157.e5
24. Weisberg E, Bateson D, McGeechan K, Mohapatra L. A three-year comparative study of continuation rates, bleeding patterns and satisfaction in Australian women using a subdermal contraceptive implant or progestogen releasing-intrauterine system. *Eur J Contracept Reprod Health Care.* 2014;19:5-14
25. Berenson AB, Tan A, Hirth JM. Complications and continuation rates associated with 2 types of long-acting contraception. *Am J Obstet Gynecol.* 2015;212(6):761.e-761.e8
26. Curtis K, Tepper N, Jatlaoui T, et al. U.S. Medical Eligibility Criteria for Contraceptive Use, 2016. *MMWR Recomm Rep.* 2016;65(3):1-103
27. American College of Obstetricians and Gynecologists Committee on Practice Bulletins-Gynecology and the Long-Acting Reversible Contraception Work Group. Practice Bulletin No. 186: Long-acting reversible contraception: implants and intrauterine devices. *Obstet Gynecol.* 2017;130(5):e251-e269
28. Braga G, Ferriolli E, Quintana S, Ferriana R, Pfrimer K, Vieira C. Immediate postpartum initiation of etonogestrel-releasing implant: a randomized controlled trial on breastfeeding impact. *Contraception.* 2015;92:536-542
29. Gurtcheff S, Turok D, Stoddard G, Murphy P, Gibson M, Jones K. Lactogenesis after early postpartum use of the contraceptive implant: a randomized controlled trial. *Obstet Gynecol.* 2011;117:1114-1121
30. Mansour D, Korver T, Marintcheva-Petrova M, Fraser IS. The effects of Implanon on menstrual bleeding patterns. *Eur J Contracept Reprod Health Care.* 2008;13(Suppl 1):13-28
31. Funk S, Miller M, Mishell DJ, et al. Safety and efficacy of Implanon, a single-rod implantable contraceptive containing etonogestrel. *Contraception.* 2005;71:319-326
32. Casey P, Long M, Marnach M, Burr J. Bleeding related to etonogestrel subdermal implant in a US population. *Contraception.* 2011;83:426-430
33. Xu H, Wade J, Peipert J, Zhao Q, Madden T, Secura G. Contraceptive failure rates of etonogestrel subdermal implants in overweight and obese women. *Obstet Gynecol.* 2012;120:21-26
34. Morrell K, Cremers S, Westhoff CL, Davis A. Relationship between etonogestrel level and BMI in women using the contraceptive implant for more than 1 year. *Contraception.* 2016;93:263-265
35. Curtis K, Jatlaoui T, Tepper N, et al. U.S. Selected Practice Recommendations for Contraceptive Use, 2016. *MMWR Recomm Rep.* 2016;65(4):1-66
36. Nexplanon. Merck & Co Inc. 2017. https://www.merckconnect.com/nexplanon/overview.html. Accessed July 10, 2018
37. Creinin M, Kaunitz A, Darney P, et al. The US etonogestrel implant mandatory clinical training and active monitoring programs: 6-year experience. *Contraception.* 2017;95:205-210

38. Guiahi M, Tocce K, Teal S, Green T, Rochon P. Removal of a Nexplanon implant located in the biceps muscle using a combination of ultrasound and fluoroscopy guidance. *Contraception.* 2014;90:606-608
39. Flore M, Chen X, Bonney A, et al. Patients' perspectives about why they have their contraceptive Implanon NXT device removed early. *Aust Fam Physician.* 2016;45(10):740-744
40. Blumenthal P, Gemzell-Danielsson K, Marintcheva-Petrova M. Tolerability and clinical safety of Implanon. *Eur J Contracept Reprod Health Care.* 2008;13(Suppl 1):29-36
41. Zigler R, McNicholas C. Unscheduled vaginal bleeding with progestin-only contraceptive use. *Am J Obstet Gynecol.* 2017;216(5):443-450
42. Phaliwong P, Taneepanichskul S. The effect of mefenamic acid on controlling irregular uterine bleeding second to Implanon use. *J Med Assoc Thai.* 2004;87(Suppl 3):S64-S68
43. Casey P, Long M, Drozdowicz L, Marnach M, Weaver A. Management of etonogestrel subdermal implant-related bleeding. *J Reprod Med.* 2014;59:306-312
44. Hou M, McNicholas C, Creinin M. Combined oral contraceptive treatment for bleeding complaints with the etonogestrel contraceptive implant: a randomised controlled trial. *Eur J Contracept Reprod Health Care.* 2016;21(5):361-366
45. Guiahi M, McBride M, Sheeder J, Teal S. Short-term treatment of bothersome bleeding for etonogestrel implant users using a 14-day oral contraceptive pill regimen: a randomized controlled trial. *Obstet Gynecol.* 2015;126:508-513
46. Weisberg E, Hickey M, Palmer D, et al. A pilot study to assess the effect of three short-term treatments on frequent and/or prolonged bleeding compared to placebo in women using Implanon. *Hum Reprod.* 2006;21:295-302
47. Weisberg E, Hickey M, Palmer D, et al. A randomized controlled trial of treatment options for troublesome uterine bleeding in Implanon users. *Hum Reprod.* 2009;24:1852-1861
48. Phupong V, Sophnsritsuk A, Taneepanichskul S. The effect of tranexamic acid for treatment of irregular uterine bleeding secondary to Norplant use. *Contraception.* 2006;73:253-256
49. Abdel-Aleem H, Shaaban O, Amin A, Abdel-Aleem A. Tamoxifen treatment of bleeding irregularities associated with Norplant use. *Contraception.* 2005;72:432-437
50. Simmons K, Edelman A, Fu R, Jensen J. Tamoxifen for the treatment of breakthrough bleeding with the etonogestrel implant: a randomized controlled trial. *Contraception.* 2017;95:198-204
51. Guazzelli C, de Queiroz F, Barbieri M, Torloni M, de Araujo F. Etonogestrel implant in adolescents: evaluation of clinical aspects. *Contraception.* 2011;83(4):336-339
52. Villas-Boas J, Vilodre L, Malerba H, et al. Metabolic safety of the etonogestrel contraceptive implant in healthy women over a 3-year period. *Eur J Obstet Gyn R B.* 2016;202:51-54
53. Guazzelli C, de Queiroz F, Barbieri M, Barreiros F, Torloni M, Araujo F. Metabolic effects of contraceptive implants in adolescents. *Contraception.* 2011;84:409-412
54. Merki-Field G, Imthurn B, Seifert B. Effects of the progestagen-only contraceptive implant Implanon on cardiovascular risk factors. *Clin Endocrinol (Oxf).* 2008;68:355-360
55. Beerthuizen R, Van Beek A, Massai R, Makarainen L, Hout J, Bennink H. Bone mineral density during long-term use of the progestagen contraceptive implant Implanon compared to a non-hormonal method of contraception. *Hum Reprod.* 2000;15:118-122
56. Bahamondes L, Monteiro-Dantas C, Espejo-Arce X, et al. A prospective study of the forearm bone density of users of etonogestrel- and levonorgestrel-releasing contraceptive implants. *Hum Reprod.* 2006;21(2):466-470
57. Chappell C, Lamorde M, Nakalema S, et al. Efavirenz decreases etonogestrel exposure: a pharmacokinetic evaluation of implantable contraception with antiretroviral therapy. *AIDS.* 2017;31:1965-1972
58. Leticee N, Viard J, Yamgnane A, Karmochkine M, Benachi A. Contraceptive failure of etonogestrel implant in patients treated with antiretrovirals including efavirenz. *Contraception.* 2012;85:425-427
59. Larorwitz A, Davis A, Swartz M, Guiahi M. The effect of carbamazepine on etonogestrel concentrations in contraceptive implant users. *Contraception.* 2017;95:571-577

60. Crouthamel B, Schiff M, Oelschlager A-MEA, Prager S, Debiec K. Bits and pieces: a crowd-sourced series of 54 cases of fractured hormonal implants. *J Pediatr Adolesc Gynecol.* 2018;31:128-131
61. Kang S, Niak A, Gada N, Brinker A, Jones S. Etonogestrel implant migration to the vasculature, chest wall, and distant body sites: cases from a pharmacovigilance database. *Contraception.* 2017;96:439-445
62. Rowlands S, Mansour D, Walling M. Intravascular migration of contraceptive implants: two more cases. *Contraception.* 2017;95:211-214
63. Gallon A, Fontarensky M, Chauffour C, Boyer L, Chabrot P. Looking for a lost subdermal contraceptive implant? Think about the pulmonary artery. *Contraception.* 2017;95:215-217
64. Chung M, Loudill C, Wieler M, Farnam J, Ahn S. Endovascular retrieval of Nexplanon from the distal pulmonary artery. *J Vasc Interv Radiol.* 2017;28(3):466-467
65. Thomas P, DiStefano D, Couteau C, D'Journo X. Contraceptive implant embolism into the pulmonary artery: thoracoscopic retrieval. *Ann Thorac Surg.* 2017;103:e271-e272
66. Barlow-Evans R, Jaffer K, Balogun M. Migration of a Nexplanon contraceptive implant to the pulmonary artery. *BMJ Case Rep.* 2017;pii:bcr-2017-219259
67. Diego D, Tappy E, Carugno J. Axillary migration of Nexplanon: case report. *Contraception.* 2017;95:218-220
68. Park J, Bae H, Lee S, Bae J, Park J. Removal of a subdermal contraceptive implant (Implanon NXT) that migrated to the axilla by C-arm guidance: a case report and review of the literature. *Medicine (Baltimore).* 2017;96(48):e8627
69. Gillies R, Scougall P, Nicklin S. Etonogestrel implants: case studies of median nerve injury following removal. *Aust Fam Physician.* 2011;40(10):799-800
70. Serati M, Bogani G, Kumar S, Cromi A, Ghezzi F. Delayed-type hypersensitivity reaction against Nexplanon. *Contraception.* 2015;91:91-92
71. Pedroso C, Martins I, Palma F, Machado A. Implant site Nexplanon reaction? *BMJ Case Rep.* 2015;pii:bcr2014206256

Adolesc Med 030 (2019) 134-149

When "Plan A" Fails: Emergency Contraception

Samuel O. Master, DO[a*]; Melanie A. Gold, DO, DMQ[b]

[a]Section of Adolescent Medicine, Department of Pediatrics, Columbia University Irving Medical Center, New York-Presbyterian Hospital, New York, New York; [b]Professor of Pediatrics, Columbia University Irving Medical Center, Professor of Population and Family Health, Mailman School of Public Health, Medical Director, School Based Health Centers, New York-Presbyterian Hospital, New York, New York

LEARNING OBJECTIVES

After reviewing this article, the reader should be able to:

1. Describe the currently available forms of oral and intrauterine emergency contraception (EC), including the advantages and disadvantages of each method
2. Differentiate between levonorgestrel, ulipristal acetate, and the copper intrauterine device (IUD) in terms of mechanism of action, overall effectiveness, and effectiveness related to timing of use, body mass index, and adverse effects
3. Explain why the copper IUD is the most effective form of EC
4. Describe how best to initiate ongoing hormonal contraception after using EC
5. Identify common barriers and solutions to patients' access to EC in a timely manner

INTRODUCTION

Emergency contraception (EC) is a safe and effective intervention that can be used postcoitally to prevent unintended pregnancy. According to the United States (US) Food and Drugs Administration (FDA) and the National Institutes of Health, pregnancy begins with uterine implantation.[1] Emergency contracep-

*Corresponding author
E-mail address: Sam.O.Master@gmail.com

 ISSN 1934-4287

tion does not cause an abortion or miscarriage, harm or dislodge an existing pregnancy,[2] or have any long-term effect on fertility.[3]

In this review article, we will discuss various forms of EC, how and when each should be used, and review myths and obstacles that discourage its use.

NEED FOR EC

The need for EC is great. In 2011, 75% of 15- to 24-year-olds, 59% of young adults, and 31% to 42% of older adults had either mistimed or unwanted pregnancies.[4,5] These pregnancies are associated with late prenatal care, reduction in breastfeeding, maternal depression, increased risk of physical violence to the mother, and financial burden.[6] The children who are born from these pregnancies are more likely to have low birth weight, more birth defects, and poor mental and physical functioning in early childhood.[7]

In 2013, 24% of pregnancies among 15- to 19-year-olds ended in abortion, while 61% resulted in live births.[8] Whereas 90% of adolescents who do not give birth during high school graduate, only 50% of teenage mothers receive a high school diploma by the age of 22 years.[9] Children born to teenage mothers are more likely to have health problems, be incarcerated, become a teenage parent themselves, have lower school achievement, and face unemployment as adults regardless of socioeconomic status.[10] In 2010, almost $9.5 billion was spent in the United States for increased health care costs and foster care, increased incarceration rates, and lost tax revenue related to teen pregnancy and childbirth.[11] With appropriate use of EC, many of these negative outcomes and costs could be avoided.

Modern contraceptives are very effective at preventing pregnancy when used correctly.[12] In 2008, two-thirds of those at risk for pregnancy who consistently used contraceptives accounted for only 5% of the unintended pregnancies. The 18% of those patients at risk for pregnancy who inconsistently used contraception accounted for 41% of the unintended pregnancies. The 14% of those at risk for pregnancy who did not use any contraception or had a gap of 1 month or longer without using contraception accounted for 54% of the unintended pregnancies.[13]

INDICATIONS

Emergency contraception is appropriate when either no contraception was used during sexual intercourse or when there was a contraceptive failure. Examples of contraceptive use failure include[14]:

- A barrier method breaks, slips, or is removed early
- Three or more combined oral contraceptive (COC) pills are consecutively missed
- Progestin-only mini-pills are taken more than 3 hours late

- The person is more than 2 weeks late receiving a depot medroxyprogesterone acetate injection
- Delay in placing or detachment of a transdermal contraceptive
- Delay in insertion or early removal of a contraceptive vaginal ring
- Failed coitus interruptus (withdrawal)
- Miscalculation of fertility cycle
- Failure of spermicide
- Expulsion of intrauterine contraception
- Having unprotected sex during the time period before an intrauterine device (IUD) or contraceptive implant is effective postinsertion

Emergency contraception may prevent up to half of all unintended pregnancies and almost three-quarters of all abortions.[15] Adolescents are less likely to use ongoing contraception and are more likely to experience sexual assault and rape-related pregnancies than adults.[16,17] Approximately 22,000 pregnancies from rape could be prevented each year with EC.[18] Among many nationally renowned academic organizations, the American Academy of Pediatrics,[19] American College of Obstetricians and Gynecologists,[20] Society for Adolescent Health and Medicine,[21] American Academy of Family Physicians,[22] and many others all recommend EC be offered to adolescents both in advance and when needed after unprotected sex.[23] Awareness of EC currently ranges from approximately 50%[24] to 95%[25] and may depend on age, access to an adolescent-specific health care center, and education level.

There are no medical conditions in which the risks of using EC outweigh the benefits of its use.[26] Although many myths are spread regarding the short- and long-term negative health outcomes of EC use (Table 1), even repeated use of EC is less harmful than pregnancy, and many studies show no safety concerns, even when EC is used more than once per menstrual cycle. Although it is not recommended to take EC frequently because of lower efficacy compared to other ongoing forms of hormonal contraception, even weekly use over the course of 2 months showed no safety issues.[27] There is also no contraindication to giving a repeat dose of hormonal EC if a second episode of unprotected intercourse follows the first administration.[28] Even with weekly EC use, there are no special safety concerns.[29] False claims about EC causing infertility and abortion[30] or causing harm when mixed with substance use are pervasive.[31] Despite these findings, studies continually prove EC to be safe.[32]

Using EC or having access to EC in advance of need does not seem to cause individuals to have unprotected sex or discontinue ongoing contraception use.[33] They do not have sex more frequently, do not have more partners, and do not have increased reported acquisition of contracting sexually transmitted infections.[34] Individuals do not use EC as a substitute method for contraception,[35,36] and EC use can even encourage individuals currently utilizing contraception to switch to more effective methods after EC use.[37] Most importantly, EC will not

Table 1
EC myths and truths

Myths	Facts
EC causes cancer	There are no scientific studies linking EC and cancer
EC causes abortions and miscarriages	EC will not affect an existing pregnancy
EC may lead to infertility	Multiple studies prove the safety of EC, even when taken repeatedly
EC is prescription only	Some forms of EC are available over-the-counter
You may only take EC once	Although EC is not as effective as long-term contraception, it may be taken frequently without health risks
All the online information about EC is medically accurate	Stories and anecdotes are frequently shared among adolescents, but it is important to trust sources with credible evidence and scientific proof
EC only works if it is taken the morning after sexual intercourse	The "morning after pill" is a nickname for some forms of EC, but it may be taken within 72-120 hours of sexual intercourse
EC encourages unprotected sex	Increased access to EC does not decrease regular contraception use or increase unprotected sex
EC is only for teenagers	EC can be used by patients of all ages
EC is only available during an emergency	Advanced provision of EC is available from medical professionals, and the Internet and can help guarantee its availability when needed
EC prevents against sexually transmitted infections	EC may help prevent a pregnancy, but it has no role in infection protection
EC is difficult to obtain	EC may be prescribed by a physician, purchased over-the-counter, or purchased online
EC is ineffective if alcohol is involved	EC is not affected by alcohol, tobacco, or other party drugs
EC is too expensive	Although a one-time fee may seem excessive, it is significantly lower than the cost of a pregnancy and is often covered by insurance or provided at a local clinic

EC, emergency contraception.

cause an abortion or cause any birth defects.[38] There is no point during the menstrual cycle when any EC available in the United States would terminate a pregnancy once implantation has occurred.[39,40] More myths regarding EC are summarized in Table 1.

TYPES OF EC

The main types of EC available in the United States are pill form and the copper IUD. The 3 different formulations for the pill are progestin-only, combined estrogen and progestin, and an antiprogestin/selective progestin receptor modulator.

No laboratory test or physical examination is needed before providing hormonal EC[32]; however, an assessment should be made regarding timing of intercourse (to ensure intercourse did not occur beyond the time at which EC is effective). This visit is an opportunity to review education about consent and discuss possible sexual assault, which would warrant further testing and support.

The use of combined oral estrogen and progestin for EC, often referred to as the Yuzpe method (after the Canadian obstetrician-gynecologist who first described the method), utilizes formulations of COC pills. A total dose of 200 mcg ethinyl estradiol and 1 mg levonorgestrel (LNG) can reduce the risk of pregnancy when taken as 2 doses 12 hours apart within 120 hours of unprotected intercourse.[41] Despite its limitations (eg, higher dose, more pills, more side effects), the Yuzpe method may still have a role in limited resource settings.[42,43] For example, in areas where EC pills are not available, COCs may be used in specific combinations for EC purposes.[44] More than 25 brands of COCs may be utilized in the United States for EC.[45] Contraindications to taking estrogen include migraines with aura, hypertension (systolic blood pressure ≥160 mm Hg or diastolic ≥100 mm Hg), known risk of thrombosis, personal history of cardiovascular disease/stroke/deep vein thrombosis, active liver disease, breast cancer, and medication interactions. These contraindications are for ongoing hormonal contraception containing estrogen and do not exist for those seeking EC.[26] The Yuzpe method of multiple COCs is the least effective EC method[46] with the most adverse effects[41] and is no longer a standard of care.

Progestin-only EC pills contain LNG (commonly referred to as Plan B). The original prescription included 1 dose of 0.75 mg LNG within 72 hours of intercourse and a second dose of 0.75 mg LNG 12 hours later. Subsequent studies proved that a single dose of 1.5 mg of LNG is just as effective as the 2-dose regimen[47] and reduced improper timing or missed administration of the second dose. Soon after the FDA approved a single-dose 1.5-mg pill taken within 72 hours of unprotected penile–vaginal intercourse for EC in 2009, the manufacturer stopped producing the 2-dose LNG EC pill formulation (Table 2 lists timing and efficacy). Levonorgestrel affects ovulation by altering luteal function with no effect on the endometrium.[48,49] It does not affect endometrial receptivity markers[50] and does not affect endometrial implantation.[51] Although a 1974 study found interference of sperm migration and function as a result of LNG,[52] a 2007 study specifically assessing this finding determined that 1.5 mg LNG does not affect sperm function or penetration of cervical mucus.[53]

The oral antiprogestin/selective progestin receptor modulators ulipristal acetate (UPA; single 30-mg dose) and mifepristone have been found to be effective forms of EC.[54] Ulipristal acetate (ella) was approved by the FDA in 2010 by prescription only (in Europe it is available over-the-counter) (Table 2 lists timing and efficacy). It inhibits ovulation, even when administered shortly before the luteinizing hormone peak, by affecting follicular development and rupture.[55] Ovulation blockade does not occur, however, once the luteinizing hormone surge peaks.[56] Some studies suggest that UPA may affect ciliary beating frequency and muscular contraction of the fallopian tube[57] without increasing the risk of ectopic pregnancy,[58] but other studies have shown no direct effect on cilia structure or function.[59] Low-dose UPA (30 mg) has no significant effect on the endometrium,[60] but different doses taken over consistent and longer periods of time were shown to affect endometrial thickness.[61] Similarly to LNG, there was no observable changes with UPA and embryo implantation.[62] In contrast to LNG, UPA may suppress the progesterone-induced acrosome reaction, hyperactivation, and calcium concentration in spermatozoa, negatively affecting sperm function through progesterone antagonism.[63]

Mifepristone is effective for EC and is approved in many countries as a medical intervention for an early first trimester abortion; it is not available in the United States as EC.[64] Mifepristone binds to progesterone receptors, blocking their effects, and prevents ovulation and endometrial development.[65] A one-time dose of 10 mg mifepristone may be given within 120 hours of unprotected penile–vaginal intercourse[66] and has equivalent efficacy to LNG.[52] A meta-analysis in 2008 found that mifepristone doses of 25 to 50 mg had lower failure rates with similar adverse effects compared to LNG.[67]

The most effective form of EC is the copper IUD.[68] One of the biggest advantages of the copper IUD is that it can be left in place to provide ongoing contraception for at least 10 years[69] and has 1-year continuation rates up to approximately 60% in individuals of all ages.[70] Contraindications for copper IUD insertion include known current infections with gonorrhea or chlamydia, mucopurulent cervicitis, pelvic inflammatory disease within the past 3 months, abnormalities of the uterus distorting the uterine cavity, postpartum endometritis or postabortal endometritis in the past 3 months, known or suspected uterine or cervical malignancy, genital bleeding of unknown etiology, Wilson disease, allergy to copper, or currently having another IUD in place.[71] An obstacle to copper IUD insertion is finding a medical professional or facility that is experienced in inserting IUDs and is available to insert the device within 5 days of unprotected intercourse. When same-day copper IUD placement was offered for EC, 11% chose the copper IUD instead of taking oral EC or returning for IUD insertion.[72] At this time, there are no confirmed trials utilizing hormonal IUDs as EC, but studies are currently evaluating their potential role.[73] Table 2 summarizes EC type by mechanism of action, timing for use, effectiveness, cost, and adverse effects.

In addition to decreasing efficacy based on timing of administration after unprotected sex (Table 2), various methods of EC have efficacy changes based on body mass index (BMI). Regardless of which oral EC was taken, there was a 3-fold greater risk for pregnancy among those who were obese (BMI $\geq$30 kg/m^2) and a 1.5 times greater risk for those who were overweight (BMI 25-30 kg/m^2).[43]

Table 2
EC type by mechanism of action, timing for use, effectiveness, cost, and adverse effects

EC type	Mechanism of action	Timing for use/ when can be used postcoitally	Effectiveness[a]	Cost[b]	Adverse effects
Levonorgestrel (Plan B, Next Choice, My Way, Take Action, Fallback Solo, e-Contra EZ, Opcicon, Aftera, React, Option 2, AfterPill)	Prevents ovulation and fertilization	Linear relationship between efficacy and time of intercourse[c] Packaging label recommends as soon as possible within 72 hours, but has reduced efficacy up to 120 hours[d] Only effective if taken before LH surge	Package insert: 88% Published literature: 52%-100%[e] Not effective once implantation or fertilization has begun[f]	Based on prescription coverage, ~$0-$60	Nausea (24%), vomiting (9%),[g] non-menstrual bleeding in the first week after use (16%),[h] and, less commonly, dizziness, fatigue, headache, breast tenderness, and lower abdominal pain[i]
Ulipristal acetate (ella)	Selective progesterone receptor modulator with primarily antiprogestin activity Postpones follicular rupture and may delay or prevent ovulation[j]	Up to 120 hours after intercourse with consistent efficacy, even after LH levels begin to rise (but not peak)[k]	No statistically significant difference from above within 72 hours of intercourse, but more effective between 72 and 120 hours[k,l] Not effective once implantation or fertilization has begun[f]	Based on prescription coverage, ~$0-$70	Headache (18%), abdominal pain (12%), nausea (12%), dysmenorrhea (9%), fatigue (6%), dizziness (5%) May reduce contraceptive action of ongoing hormonal contraceptive[m]

Copper IUD (ParaGard)	Prevents fertilization through the effect of copper ions on sperm function If fertilization has occurred, copper ions prevent endometrial receptivity[n]	Up to 120 hours after ovulation, but because of difficulty determining exact day of ovulation through history, recommended for up to 120 hours after intercourse[o]	>99% effective[p]	Based on prescription coverage, 0-$800	Dysmenorrhea, vaginal bleeding, leukorrhea, vasovagal reaction, expulsion of device, dyspareunia, PID if infection present during time of insertion

EC, emergency contraception; IUD, intrauterine device; LH, luteinizing hormone; PID, pelvic inflammatory disease.

[a] Effectiveness is difficult to measure because of the lack of randomized control trials in comparison to placebo.

[b] Cost depends on insurance, access to Title X-funded sites, and funding to Title X sites.

[c] Piaggio G, von Hertzen H, Grimes DA, Van Look PF. Timing of emergency contraception with levonorgestrel or the Yuzpe regimen. Task Force on Postovulatory Methods of Fertility Regulation. *Lancet*. 1999;353(9154):721.

[d] Piaggio G, Kapp N, von Hertzen H. Effect on pregnancy rates of the delay in the administration of levonorgestrel for emergency contraception: a combined analysis of 4 WHO trials. *Contraception*. 2011;84(1):35:39.

[e] Trussell J, Raymond EG. Emergency contraception: a last chance to prevent unintended pregnancy. November 2011. http://ec.princeton.edu/questions/ec-review.pdf. Accessed May 24, 2018

[f] Trussell J, Jordan B. Mechanism of action of emergency contraceptive pills. *Contraception*. 2006;74(2):87-89.

[g] Rodriguez MI, Godfrey EM, Warden M, Curtis KM. Prevention and management of nausea and vomiting with emergency contraception: a systematic review. *Contraception*. 2013;87(5):583-589.

[h] Kesseru E, Gardmendia F, Westphal N, Parada J. The hormonal and peripheral effects of d-norgestrel in postcoital contraception. *Contraception*. 1974;10(4):411-424.

[i] Practice Bulletin No. 152: Emergency contraception. *Obstet Gynecol*. 2015;126(3):e1-311. Reaffirmed 2018.

[j] Gemzell-Danielsson K, Berger C, Lalitkumar PGL. Emergency contraception—mechanisms of action. *Contraception*. 2013;87(3):300-308.

[k] Glasier AF, Cameron ST, Fine PM, et al. Ulipristal acetate versus levonorgestrel for emergency contraception: a randomised non-inferiority trial and meta-analysis. *Lancet*. 2010;375(9714):555-562.

[l] Creinin MD, Schlaff W, Archer DF, et al. Progesterone receptor modulator for emergency contraception: a randomized controlled trial. *Obstet Gynecol*. 2006;108(5):1089-1097.

[m] ella Prescribing Information. Afaxys Pharma, LLC, Charleston, South Carolina. September 2017

[n] Koyama A, Hagopian L, Linden J. Emerging options for emergency contraception. *Clin Med Insights Reprod Health*. 2013;7(3547):23-35

[o] Curtis KM, Tepper NK, Jatlaoui TC, et al. U.S. Medical Eligibility Criteria for Contraceptive Use, 2016. *MMWR Recomm Rep*. 2016;65(3):1-103

[p] ParaGard package insert. Trumbill, CT: Cooper Surgical; 2018

Additionally, those who were obese and taking LNG for EC had a higher rate of pregnancy than those who were obese and taking UPA for EC.[74,75] Levonorgestrel is less efficacious with increasing BMI (less effective with BMI 25-30, not proven to be effective with BMI ≥30), UPA is more efficacious than LNG with increasing BMI (equally effective as LNG with BMI 25-30, more effective than LNG for BMI ≥30, not proven to be effective with BMI ≥35), and there is no decrease in effectiveness of the copper IUD by BMI.[76] Thus, the copper IUD is the most effective choice for EC among adolescents and adults who are obese or overweight.

Although the copper IUD is useful for EC and is immediately effective for contraception,[71] oral EC can affect the efficacy of other forms of hormonal contraception because of interacting mechanisms of action. Therefore, resumption of ongoing contraception depends on which method of EC is used.[77] After LNG or a combined estrogen-progestin EC is taken, any contraceptive method can be immediately restarted, but additional barrier methods are necessary for the first week until the newly initiated ongoing contraceptive method becomes effective at suppressing ovulation.[26] Although not currently approved for EC, the LNG IUD has been preferred by some adolescents and adults when given at the same time as oral LNG EC compared to the copper IUD.[78] In comparison, UPA may be negatively influenced by hormonal contraception, making both the EC and long-term contraception less effective.[26] New studies show that the effectiveness of UPA is significantly reduced when COCs are taken 2 days later.[79] Therefore, it is generally recommended to delay starting short-acting hormonal contraception, such as the combination pills, patch, ring, or depot medroxyprogesterone acetate injections, for 5 days after the use of UPA and to use a backup method for 12 days.[26] If there is concern about follow-up, a hormonal method may be started at the same time, with counseling regarding decreased efficacy and use of barrier methods or abstinence for 7 days or until the next menstrual period.[80] There is no concern or need for reinitiating contraception after copper IUD placement.

EC ACCESS

After much litigation, the US FDA made LNG EC available over-the-counter for consumers of all ages and genders in 2013,[81] and in 2016 this availability became applicable for generic versions as well.[82] Ulipristal acetate was approved by the FDA in 2010 by prescription only,[83] but it is available over-the-counter in Europe. Both oral ECs are available online (with medical evaluations and physician review available when applicable); however, access to EC is an ongoing concern among medical professionals, pharmacists, and consumers. Some pediatricians believe that access to EC encourages risk-taking behaviors, and others have been concerned about teratogenic effects.[84] Even when appropriately prescribed, patients often have difficulty obtaining EC medication.[85] Fewer than 10% of US pharmacies could immediately fill a prescription[86] and most stated that they could order the medication, with a wait time of approximately 24 hours. Studies have shown that pharmacy access to EC changes based on the socioeconomic status of the neighborhood, the hours of operation of particular pharmacies, and the gender of the individual trying to purchase EC.[87] Many emergency departments do not provide EC, even in situations of sexual assault and rape, even though they have legal responsibilities to provide such care.[88-90] Individuals are concerned about confidentiality, possible adverse effects, and transportation required to acquire EC medication,[91] but, regardless of gender, are interested in obtaining EC when available.[92] Fewer than 20% of college-aged students were aware that EC was available in their local health center,[93] and some universities are trying to increase access to EC with vending machines.[94] Persistent barriers exist, such as pharmacists who have refused to dispense EC based on the gender and age of the patient either in person or over the phone, but in some states (eg, Alaska, California, Hawaii, Maine, Massachusetts, New Hampshire, New Mexico, Vermont, and Washington[95]), pharmacists actually increase care by prescribing and providing EC.[96]

In an effort to increase access, oral EC is now available online for purchase. At the time of this publication, oral LNG is available on Web sites such as www.afterpill.com, www.amazon.com, and online pharmacies (CVS.com, RiteAid.com, Target.com, Walgreens.com, Walmart.com, Drugstore.com) with expedited and standard shipping options available and prices comparable to purchasing in person. Ulipristal acetate may also be purchased online through Web sites such as www.kiwmed.com and their partner www.prjktruby.com, from which a licensed US physician can review the order and, if deemed appropriate, prescribe UPA, which arrives in discreet packaging and requires a signature on delivery, with next-day delivery coupons available on www.ellanow.com. Some Web sites, occasionally state-specific, include health questionnaires, online consultations, and insurance information (for reduced costs), such as https://app.nurx.co, https://thepillclub.com, www.pandiahealth.com, and www.mavenclinic.com, to help facilitate access to EC. Advanced provision of EC for individuals, although not proven to decrease pregnancy,[97] has a positive effect on the use and timing of EC and does not negatively affect contraceptive use or sexual risk-taking behaviors.[98]

CONCLUSION

Emergency contraception is a safe and effective intervention that can be used postcoitally to prevent unintended pregnancy. It has the potential to prevent up to half of all unintended pregnancies and almost three-quarters of all abortions, and it can be used when either no contraception was used during sexual intercourse or there was a contraceptive failure.

The main types of EC available in the United States are pill form (LNG, UPA) and the copper IUD. The copper IUD is the most efficacious EC method, followed by UPA and LNG. The efficacy of the copper IUD is not affected by the timing of unprotected intercourse, BMI, or medication interactions.

Many barriers still exist to obtaining EC, despite legal rulings and access to EC through the Internet. Better and more accurate information for prescription writers, fillers, and patients will help facilitate efficient and appropriate use of this necessary medication for those who require and warrant its use.

QUESTIONS

1. A 16-year-old female with a body mass index (BMI) of 39 kg/m^2 comes to your office 4 days after unprotected penile–vaginal intercourse and wishes to avoid pregnancy. Which is the most effective emergency contraception (EC) option for her at this time?
   A. Oral levonorgestrel
   B. Oral ulipristal acetate
   C. Copper intrauterine device (IUD)
   D. They are all equally effective
2. You are seeing an 18-year-old transgender male for his college physical examination, and he asks you how to get EC if necessary while he is away at school. What can you tell him?
   A. He can buy over-the-counter levonorgestrel when he needs it.
   B. He can get a prescription from his college health service.
   C. You can give him an advanced prescription for later use.
   D. He can order EC over the Internet when he needs it.
   E. All of the above
3. A 17-year-old male comes into your office for a sports physical, and he tells you he is upset because his condom broke last night when he was having sexual intercourse with his girlfriend. He doesn't feel ready to be a father. How can you best help him address last night's contraceptive failure?
   A. Tell him to stop having sex from now on.
   B. Advise him to tell his girlfriend to come into the office for EC.
   C. Offer him sexually transmitted infection (STI) and human immunodeficiency virus testing today.
   D. Give him EC to give to his girlfriend.
   E. Teach him how to use condoms correctly so that it does not happen again.

(See pages 202-203 for answers.)

References

1. Protection of Human Subjects, 45 CFR Section 46.202. 2009. https://www.hhs.gov/ohrp/regulations-and-policy/regulations/regulatory-text/index.html#46.202. Accessed May 25, 2018
2. Levonorgestrel for emergency contraception. Fact sheet. Geneva, Switzerland: World Health Organization; 2005
3. Glasier A. Emergency postcoital contraception. *N Engl J Med.* 1997;337:1058-1064

4. Finer LB, Zolna MR. Declines in unintended pregnancy in the United States, 2008–2011. *N Engl J Med.* 2016;374(9):843-852
5. Satterwhite CL, Torrone E, Meites E, et al. Sexually transmitted infections among US women and men: prevalence and incidence estimates, 2008. *Sex Transm Dis.* 2013;40:187-193
6. Singh S, Sedgh G, Hussain R. Unintended pregnancy: worldwide levels, trends, and outcomes. *Stud Fam Plann.* 2010;41:241-250
7. Conde-Agudelo A, Rosas-Bermúdez A, Kafury-Goeta AC. Effects of birth spacing on maternal health: a systematic review. *Am J Obstet Gynecol.* 2007;196:297-308
8. Kost K, Maddow-Zimet I, Arpaia A. *Pregnancies, Births and Abortions Among Adolescents and Young Women in the United States, 2013: National and State Trends by Age, Race and Ethnicity.* New York: Guttmacher Institute; 2017
9. Perper K, Peterson K, Manlove J. *Diploma Attainment Among Teen Mothers. Child Trends.* Fact Sheet Publication #2010-01. Washington, DC: Child Trends; 2010
10. Hoffman SD. *Kids Having Kids: Economic Costs and Social Consequences of Teen Pregnancy.* Washington, DC: The Urban Institute Press; 2008
11. National Campaign to Prevent Teen and Unplanned Pregnancy. Counting it up: the public costs of teen childbearing 2013. https://powertodecide.org/what-we-do/information/resource-library/counting-it-key-data. Accessed June 18, 2018
12. Trussell J. Contraceptive failure in the United States. *Contraception.* 2011;83(5):397-404
13. Sonfield A, Hasstedt K, Gold RB. *Moving Forward, Family Planning in the Era of Health Reform,* New York: Guttmacher Institute, 2014
14. World Health Organization Fact Sheet No. 244. Emergency contraception. 2018. http://www.who.int/news-room/fact-sheets/detail/emergency-contraception. Accessed June 18, 2018
15. Trussell J, Stewart F, Guest F, et al. Emergency contraceptive pills: a simple proposal to reduce unintended pregnancies. *Fam Plann Perspect.* 1992;24:269-273
16. Crawford-Jakubiak JE, Alderman EM, Leventhal JM; American Academy of Pediatrics Committee on Child Abuse and Neglect. Care of the adolescent after an acute sexual assault. *Pediatrics.* 2017;*139*(3):e20164243
17. Wilson F, Klein J. Opportunities for appropriate care: health care and contraceptive use among adolescents reporting unwanted sexual intercourse. *Arch Pediatr Adolesc Med.* 2002;156:341-344
18. Stewart FH, Trussell J. Prevention of pregnancy resulting from rape: a neglected preventive health measure. *Am J Prev Med.* 2000;19:228-229
19. American Academy of Pediatrics Committee on Adolescence. Emergency contraception. *Pediatrics.* 2012;130(6):1174-1182
20. American College of Obstetricians and Gynecologists Committee on Health Care for Underserved Women. ACOG Committee Opinion No. 707: Access to emergency contraception. *Obstet Gynecol.* 2017;130:e48-e52
21. Society for Adolescent Health and Medicine. Emergency contraception for adolescents and young adults: guidance for health care professionals. *J Adolesc Health.* 2016;58(2):245-248
22. Bosworth M, Olusola P, Low SB. An update on emergency contraception. *Am Fam Physician.* 2014;89(7):545-550
23. Whittaker, P. G., Armstrong, K. A., Adams, J. Implementing an advance emergency contraception policy: What happens in the real world? *Perspect Sex Reprod Health.* 2008;40(3):162-170
24. Ahern R, Frattarelli LA, Delto J, Kaneshiro B. Knowledge and awareness of emergency contraception in adolescents. *J Pediatr Adolesc Gynecol.* 2010;23(5):273-278
25. Aiken AM, Gold MA, Parker AM. Changes in young women's awareness, attitudes, and perceived barriers to using emergency contraception. *J Pediatr Adolesc Gynecol.* 2005;18(1):25-32
26. Curtis KM, Tepper NK, Jatlaoui TC, et al. U.S. Medical Eligibility Criteria for Contraceptive Use, 2016. *MMWR Recomm Rep.* 2016;65(3):1-103
27. Jesam C, Cochon L, Salvatierra AM, et al. A prospective, open-label, multicenter study to assess the pharmacodynamics and safety of repeated use of 30 mg ulipristal acetate. *Contraception.* 2016;93(4):310-316
28. Rowlands S, Devalia H, Lawrenson R, et al. Repeated use of hormonal emergency contraception by younger women in the UK. *Br J Fam Plann.* 2000;26(3):138–43

29. Jatlaoui TC, Riley H, Curtis KM. Safety data for levonorgestrel, ulipristal acetate and Yuzpe regimens for emergency contraception. *Contraception*. 2016;93:93-212
30. Mawathe A. Kenya concern over pill popping. BBC News. July 15, 2009. http://news.bbc.co.uk/2/hi/africa/8145418.stm. Accessed June 21, 2018
31. Khadr SN, Jones KG, Mann S, et al. Investigating the relationship between substance use and sexual behaviour in young people in Britain: findings from a national probability survey. *BMJ Open*. 2016;6(6):e011961
32. American College of Obstetricians and Gynecologists. ACOG Practice Bulletin No. 152: Emergency contraception. *Obstet Gynecol*. 2015;126(3):e1-e11. Reaffirmed 2018
33. Lo SS, Fan SY, Ho PC, Glasier AF. Effect of advanced provision of emergency contraception on women's contraceptive behaviour: a randomized controlled trial. *Hum Reprod*. 2004;19(10):2404-2410
34. Raine TR, Harper CC, Rocca CH, et al. Direct access to emergency contraception through pharmacies and effect on unintended pregnancy and STIs: a randomized controlled trial. *JAMA*. 2005;293(1):54-62
35. Blanchard K, Haskell S, Ferden S, et al. Differences between emergency contraception users in the United States and the United Kingdom. *J Am Med Womens Assoc*. 2002;57(4):200-203, 214
36. Abuabara K, Becker D, Ellertson C, Blanchard K, Schiavon R, Garcia SG. As often as needed: appropriate use of emergency contraceptive pills. *Contraception*. 2004;69(4):339-342
37. Breitbart V, Castle MA, Walsh K, Casanova C. The impact of patient experience on practice: the acceptability of emergency contraceptive pills in inner-city clinics. *J Am Med Womens Assoc*. 1998;53(5 Suppl 2):255-257, 265
38. Zhang L, Chen J, Wang Y, Ren F, Yu W, Cheng L. Pregnancy outcome after levonorgestrel-only emergency contraception failure: a prospective cohort study. *Hum Reprod*. 2009;24:1605-1611
39. Noé G, Croxatto HB, Salvatierra AM, et al. Contraceptive efficacy of emergency contraception with levonorgestrel given before or after ovulation. *Contraception*. 2011;84(5):486-492
40. Li HW, Lo SS, Ng EH, Ho PC. Efficacy of ulipristal acetate for emergency contraception and its effect on the subsequent bleeding pattern when administered before or after ovulation. *Hum Reprod*. 2016;31:1200-1207
41. Randomised controlled trial of levonorgestrel versus the Yuzpe regimen of combined oral contraceptives for emergency contraception. Task Force on Postovulatory Methods of Fertility Regulation. *Lancet*. 1998;352(9):428-433
42. Farajkhoda T, Khoshbin A, Enjezab B, et al. Assessment of two emergency contraceptive regimens in Iran: levonorgestrel versus the Yuzpe. *Niger J Clin Pract*. 2009;12:450-452
43. Glasier A, Cameron ST, Blithe D, et al. Can we identify women at risk of pregnancy despite using emergency contraception? Data from randomized trials of ulipristal acetate and levonorgestrel. *Contraception*. 2011;84(4):363-367
44. Ellertson C, Webb A, Blanchard K, et al. Modifying the Yuzpe regimen of emergency contraception: a multicenter randomized, controlled trial. *Obstet Gynecol*. 2003;101:1160-1167
45. Arowojolu AO, Okewole IA, Adekunle AO. Comparative evaluation of the effectiveness and safety of two regimens of levonorgestrel for emergency contraception in Nigerians. *Contraception*. 2002;66:269-273. Erratum in *Contraception*. 2003;67(2):165
46. Raymond E, Taylor D, Trussell J, Steiner MJ. Minimum effectiveness of the levonorgestrel regimen of emergency contraception. *Contraception*. 2004;69(1):79-81
47. von Hertzen H, Piaggio G, Ding J, et al. Low dose mifepristone and two regimens of levonorgestrel for emergency contraception: a WHO multicentre randomised trial. *Lancet*. 2002;360:1803-1810
48. Hapangama D, Glasier AF, Baird DT. The effects of peri-ovulatory administration of levonorgestrel on the menstrual cycle. *Contraception*. 2001;63:123-129
49. Durand M, del Carmen Cravioto M, Raymond EG, et al. On the mechanisms of short-term levonorgestrel administration in emergency contraception. *Contraception*. 2011;64(4):227-234
50. Meng CX, Andersson KL Bentin-Ley U, Gemzell-Danielsson K, Latilkumar PG. Effect of levonorgestrel and mifepristone on endometrial receptor activity markers in a three-dimensional human endometrial cell culture model. *Fertil Steril*. 2009;91(1):256-264

51. Lalitkumar PG, Lalitkumar S, Meng CX, et al. Mifepristone, but not levonorgestrel, inhibits human blastocyst attachment to an in vitro endometrial cell culture model. *Hum Reprod.* 2007;22(1):3031-3037
52. Kesseru E, Gardmendia F, Westphal N, Parada J. The hormonal and peripheral effects of d-norgestrel in postcoital contraception. *Contraception.* 1974;10(4):411-424
53. Do Nascimento JA, Seppala M, Perdigao A, et al. In vivo assessment of the human sperm acrosome reaction and the expression of glycodelin A in human endometrium after levonorgestrel emergency contraceptive pill administration. *Hum Reprod.* 2007;22(8):2190-2195
54. Glasier AF, Cameron ST, Fine PM, et al. Ulipristal acetate versus levonorgestrel for emergency contraception: a randomised non-inferiority trial and meta-analysis. *Lancet.* 2010;375(9714):555-562
55. Jamin C. Emergency contraception: efficacy difference between levonorgestrel and ulipristal acetate depending on the follicular size at the time of an unprotected sexual intercourse. *Gynecol Obstet Fertil.* 2015;43(3):242-247
56. Brache V, Cochon L, Jesam C, et al. Immediate pre-ovulatory administration of 30 mg ulipristal acetate significantly delays follicular rupture. *Hum Reprod.* 2010;25(9):2256-2263
57. Li HW, Liao SB, Yeung WS, Ng EH, O WS, Ho PC. Ulipristal acetate resembles mifepristone in modulating human Fallopian tube function. *Hum Reprod.* 2014;29(10):2156-2162
58. Levy DP, Jager M, Kapp N, Abitbol JL. Ulipristal acetate for emergency contraception: postmarketing experience after use by more than 1 million women. *Contraception.* 2014;89(5):431-433
59. Yuan J, Zhao W, Yan M, et al. Ulipristal acetate antagonizes the inhibitory effect of progesterone on ciliary beat frequency and upregulates steroid expression levels in human Fallopian tubes. *Reprod Sci.* 2015;22(12):1516-1523
60. Gemzell-Danielsson K, Berger C, Lalitkumar PG. Mechanisms of action of oral emergency contraception. *Gynecol Endocrinol.* 2014;30(10):685-687
61. Donnez J, Tomaszewski J, Vázquez F, et al; PEARL I Study Group. Ulipristal acetate versus leuprolide acetate for uterine fibroids. *N Engl J Med.* 2012;366(5):421-432
62. Berger C, Boggavarapu NR, Menezes J, Lalitkumar PGL, Gemzell-Danielsson K. Effects of ulipristal acetate on human embryo attachment and endometrial cell gene expression in an in vitro co-culture system. *Hum Reprod.* 2015;30(4):800-811
63. Ko JKY, Huang VW, Li RHW, Yeung WSB, Ho PC, Chiu PCN. An in vitro study of the effect of mifepristone and ulipristal acetate on human sperm functions. *Andrology.* 2014;2(6):868-874
64. Shen J, Che Y, Showell E, Chen K, Cheng L. Interventions for emergency contraception. *Cochrane Database Syst Rev.* 2017;8:CD001324
65. Wu S, Wang C, Wang Y, et al. A randomized, double blind, multicenter study on comparing levonorgestrel and mifepristone for emergency contraception. *J Reprod Med.* 1999;8(Suppl 1):S43-S46
66. Comparison of three single doses of mifepristone as emergency contraception: a randomized trial. Task Force on Postovulatory Methods of Fertility Regulation. *Lancet.* 1999;353(9154):697-702
67. Chen L, Gulmezoglu AM, Piaggio GGP, Ezcurra EE, Van Look PPFA. Interventions for emergency contraception. *Cochrane Database Syst Rev.* 2008;2:CD001324
68. Wu S, Godfrey EM, Wojdyla D, et al. Copper T380A intrauterine device for emergency contraception: a prospective, multicentre, cohort clinical trial. *BJOG.* 2010;117(10):1205-1210
69. Long-term reversible contraception. Twelve years of experience with the TCu380A and TCu220C. *Contraception.* 1997;56(6):341-352
70. Sanders JN, Turok DK, Royer PA, Thompson IS, Gawron LM, Storck KE. One-year continuation of copper or levonorgestrel intrauterine devices initiated at the time of emergency contraception. *Contraception.* 2017;96(2):99-105
71. ParaGard package insert. Trumbill, CT; Cooper Surgical, 2018
72. Schwarz EB, Papic M, Parisi SM, et al. Routine counseling about intrauterine contraception for women seeking emergency contraception. *Contraception.* 2014;90(1):66-71
73. McNicholas C, Biggs L. Levonorgestrel Intrauterine System for Emergency Contraception (LIFE). https://clinicaltrials.gov/ct2/show/NCT00995150. Accessed June 25, 2018

74. Creinin MD, Schlaff W, Archer DF, et al. Progesterone receptor modulator for emergency contraception: a randomized controlled trial. *Obstet Gynecol.* 2006;108(5):1089-1097
75. Fine P, Mathé H, Ginde S, Cullins V, Morfesis J, Gainer E. Ulipristal acetate taken 48-120 hours after intercourse for emergency contraception. *Obstet Gynecol.* 2010;115(2 Pt 1):257-263
76. Reproductive Health Technologies Project. Frequently asked questions: the impact of weight on efficacy of emergency contraception. 2013. http://rhtp.org/work/contraception/emergency-contraception/. Accessed June 25, 2018
77. Salcedo J, Rodriguez MI, Curtis KM, Kapp N. When can a woman resume or initiate contraception after taking emergency contraceptive pills? A systematic review. *Contraception.* 2013;87(5): 602-604
78. Turok DK, Sanders JN, Thompson IS, Royer PA, Eggebroten J, Gawron LM. Preference for and efficacy of oral levonorgestrel for emergency contraception with concomitant placement of a levonorgestrel IUD: a prospective cohort study. *Contraception.* 2016;93(6):526-532
79. Edelman AB, Jensen JT, McCrimmon S, et al. Combined oral contraceptive interference with the ability of ulipristal acetate to delay ovulation: a prospective cohort study. *Contraception.* 2018;98(6):463-466
80. World Health Organization. *Medical Eligibility Criteria for Contraceptive Use.* 5th ed. Geneva, Switzerland: World Health Organization, 2015
81. Department of Health and Human Services, Food and Drug Administration. DA/ANDA applicant letter. February 24, 2014. https://www.accessdata.fda.gov/drugsatfda_docs/nda/2013/021998Orig1s002.pdf. Accessed June 21, 2018
82. Korman order. Tummino v. Hamburg. Memorandum available at https://www.scribd.com/document/147599477/Korman-Order. Accessed June 25, 2018
83. US Food and Drug Administration. FDA approves ella tablets for prescription emergency contraception. https://www.accessdata.fda.gov/drugsatfda_docs/label/2010/022474s000lbl.pdf. Accessed June 25, 2018
84. Golden NH, Seigel WM, Fisher M, et al. Emergency contraception: pediatricians' knowledge, attitudes, and opinions. *Pediatrics.* 2001;107(2):287-292
85. Simonds W, Ellertson C. Emergency contraception and morality: reflections of health care workers and clients. *Soc Sci Med.* 2004;58(7):1285-1297
86. Shigesato M, Elia J, Tschann M, et al. Pharmacy access to Ulipristal acetate in major cities throughout the United States. *Contraception.* 2018;97(3):264-269
87. Bell DL, Camacho EJ, Velasquez AB. Male access to emergency contraception in pharmacies: a mystery shopper survey. *Contraception.* 2014;90(4):413-415
88. Patel A, Panchal H, Piotrowski ZH, Patel D. Comprehensive medical care for victims of sexual assault: a survey of Illinois hospital emergency departments. *Contraception.* 2008;77(6):426-430
89. Kavanaugh ML, Saladino RA, Gold MA. Emergency contraception services for adolescents: a national survey of Children's Hospital Emergency Department Directors. *J Pediatr Adolesc Gynecol.* 2009;22(2):111-119
90. Goldenring JM, Allred G. Post-rape care in hospital emergency rooms. *Am J Public Health.* 2001;91(8):1169-1170
91. Mollen CJ, Barg FK, Hayes KL, et al. Assessing attitudes about emergency contraception among urban, minority adolescent girls: an in-depth interview study. *Pediatrics.* 2008;122(2):e395-e401
92. Garbers S, Bell DL, Ogaye K, Marcell AV, Westhoff CL, Rosenthal SL. Advance provision of emergency contraception to young men: an exploratory study in a clinic setting. *Contraception.* 2018;98(2):106-109
93. Miller LM. College student knowledge and attitudes toward emergency contraception. *Contraception.* 2011;83(1):68-73
94. Caron C. Students look to vending machines for better access to morning after pill. *The New York Times.* September 28, 2017
95. The Emergency Contraception Website. The Office of Population Research at Princeton University. http://ec.princeton.edu/questions/state-pharmacy-access-list.html. Updated September 5, 2017. Accessed May 24th, 2018

96. Rafie S, Stone RH, Wilkinson TA, et al. Role of the community pharmacist in emergency contraception counseling and delivery in the United States: current trends and future prospects. *Integr Pharm Res Pract*. 2017;6:99-108
97. Polis CB, Grimes DA, Schaffer K, et al. Advance provision of emergency contraception for pregnancy prevention. *Cochrane Database Syst Rev*. 2007;2:CD005497
98. Meyer JL, Gold MA, Haggerty CL. Advance provision of emergency contraception among adolescent and young adult women: a systematic review of literature. *J Pediatr Adolesc Gynecol*. 2011;24(1):2-9

Adolesc Med 030 (2019) 150–160

Implementation of LARC Methods Into Pediatric Practice

Shamieka Virella Dixon, MD

Atrium Health's Levine Children's Hospital, Teen Health Connection, Assistant Professor of Pediatrics, Charlotte, North Carolina

LEARNING OBJECTIVES

After reviewing this article, the reader should be able to:

1. Identify opportunities for further training in LARC methods
2. Navigate clinical and procedural logistics needed to implement LARC methods in practice
3. Manage common adverse effects and complications of LARC placement

INTRODUCTION

Two types of long-acting reversible contraceptives (LARCs) are available in the United States (US): intrauterine devices (IUDs) and contraceptive implants. Use of LARC for all women in the United States has increased in the past decade, from 2.4% in 2002, to 8.5% in 2009, to 11.6% in 2012. Of the 11.6% women who rely on LARC methods, 10.3% use IUDs and 1.3% use the implant.[1] However, LARC usage among adolescents remains low, with only 4% to 7% of 15- to 19-year-old females reporting use in 2012 to 2013.[2] Reducing barriers to LARC access for adolescent and young adult women may continue to lower the US unintended pregnancy rate. Pediatricians and adolescent medicine specialists are uniquely positioned to discuss contraception and pregnancy prevention with adolescents, but we must first start with intentionally counseling about these highly effective contraceptive methods and becoming certified to provide them.

E-mail address: Shamieka.Dixon@atriumhealth.org

 ISSN 1934-4287

Lack of availability of clinicians to perform on-site insertion presents a significant barrier to LARC use in adolescents who often do not follow through with referrals to specialists outside of their medical home.[3] LARC methods are more effective than traditional combined oral contraceptives (COCs) and are recommended as a first-line contraceptive choice for adolescents by the American Academy of Pediatrics and the American College of Obstetrics and Gynecology.[4,5]

TRAINING FOR IUD AND IMPLANT INSERTION

To increase adolescents' access to implants and IUDs, more pediatricians must become trained to provide these services. Of note, in accordance with US Food and Drug Administration (FDA) requirements, Merck requires clinicians (ie, physicians, physician assistants, nurse practitioners) to complete their training sessions on implant (Nexplanon) insertion and removal before they are added to Merck's list of credentialed providers who can order their product. For IUD placement, no training is required by the FDA, so clinicians must seek training on their own.

LARC Training During Residency

Pediatric residency programs provide the perfect opportunity to begin training physicians in IUD and implant placement. Some programs require pediatric residents to participate in Merck's implant training while also allowing elective time to train with physicians who place IUDs and implants in practice, if desired. Other programs have begun offering LARC placement to adolescents when they are hospitalized for various reasons, provided they meet applicable criteria and the procedure is covered by insurance. One study found that although 56% of enrolled adolescents had received primary care from a pediatrician, those adolescents had lower odds of using LARC compared to those with a family physician as their primary care physician.[2] Seventy-five percent of adolescents with a family medicine clinician had one who was credentialed in LARC methods, whereas only 8.2% of adolescents with a pediatric clinician had one who was credentialed.[2] Adolescents in this study whose primary care clinician was credentialed in LARC methods or was a resident physician had higher odds of using a LARC method.[2] Residents and fellows interested in additional experience in placing IUDs and implants may consider pursuing elective training with clinics providing LARC, such as their adolescent medicine divisions, obstetrician/gynecology practices, family planning clinics, Planned Parenthood, health departments, or other Title X-funded clinics. IUD insertions, compared to implant insertions, require more practical experience to gain competency with equipment and procedural technique. It is important that we invest in our future physicians by providing them with training during residency so that they are prepared to offer their patients access to this highly effective contraception and further reduce teen pregnancy rates.

LARC Training After Residency

For physicians who have already completed their residency and fellowship training and are interested in becoming credentialed in LARC insertion methods, many opportunities are available. Table 1 lists several reproductive health organizations and pharmaceutical companies that offer training for physicians and other primary care providers in LARC insertion methods. As noted previously, Merck training is required before ordering and placing their subdermal implant, and representatives from the company can help connect practicing physicians with a training session. Pharmaceutical representatives can also facilitate office training related to IUDs with videos and demonstration models. Training sessions are often available at national meetings of organizations that provide reproductive health care to adolescent and young adult women.

After completion of any of the classroom-based trainings, the next step is to arrange for hands-on clinical experience in placement and removal of IUDs or implants. This may require some creative scheduling for practicing physicians. Physicians should consider contacting practices affiliated with their home institution or clinical network that offer LARC methods. These practices may be able to consolidate placement or removal procedures on specific days to maximize training opportunities. Intrauterine device insertions and implants removals require

Table 1
Organizations and pharmaceutical companies that offer LARC training

ACOG LARC Program	https://www.acog.org/About-ACOG/ACOG-Departments/Long-Acting-Reversible-Contraception/LARC-Program-Activities
Association of Reproductive Health Professional (ARHP)	www.arhp.org
Contraceptive Technology	www.contraceptivetechnology.org/conferences/
National Clinical Training Center for Family Planning	www.ctcfp.org/larc/
Reproductive Health Access Project	https://www.reproductiveaccess.org/programs/hartcenter/
The Society of Family Planning	https://www.societyfp.org/Meetings-and-events/Calendar-of-events.aspx
UCSF Beyond the Pill	http://beyondthepill.ucsf.edu/site-training
Upstream	http://upstream.org
Bayer HealthCare Pharmaceuticals (Mirena, Kyleena, Skyla)	http://hcp.mirena-us.com/, https://hcp.kyleena-us.com/, http://www.skyla-us.com/index.php
Medicines360 (Liletta)	https://www.lilettahcp.com/request-a-rep
Merck & Co., Inc (Nexplanon)	https://www.nexplanontraining.com/request-clinical-training/in-person-training/
Teva Women's Health, Inc (ParaGard)	https://hcp.paragard.com/

LARC, long-acting reversible contraceptive.

more practical experience to obtain competency with the equipment, procedural techniques, and navigation through difficult insertions or removals. Some adolescent medicine programs have partnered with obstetrician/gynecology departments to have an on-site gynecologist work in the adolescent medicine clinic, thereby providing access to LARC as well as supervising training.

Hospital Credentialing

Many hospital systems require observation placing and removing a certain number of implants or IUDs by a credentialed provider before adding this new skill to one's delineation of privileges (DOP) (this process may differ for private practices). Residents and fellows trained in placing IUDs or implants should remember to add these skills to their DOP when starting a new job. They may be required to supply a patient log and provide the dates on which training was completed. It is important to add IUD and implant placement and removal to the new institution's DOP to allow for practice independence and liability coverage.

PREPARING A PRACTICE FOR LARC PLACEMENTS

Confidentiality and Staff Training

Federal regulations allow teens to seek confidential contraceptive services from Medicaid or Title X providers; however, regulations on parental consent for teens generally vary from state to state (for additional discussion see article on policy foundations supporting adolescent access to contraceptive care by Grubb and Upadhya in this issue of AM:STARs) and can also differ for those with private insurance.[6] The Guttmacher Institute (https://www.guttmacher.org) maintains up-to-date information on state minor consent laws and access to contraceptive services. It is important to establish best practices and protocols for clinical staff regarding contraceptive counseling, pregnancy, and sexually transmitted infection (STI) testing before placement, insertion techniques, equipment setup, and obtaining informed consent. Consider having prepackaged kits containing equipment needed for procedures, required consent forms, and patient care instructions. The Reproductive Health Access Project has LARC fact sheets and aftercare instructions that can be given to patients after the procedure (https://www.reproductiveaccess.org).

Procedure Appointments and Patient Access

Many practices allow for 20- or 30-minute procedure appointments, although more or less time may be needed depending on the specific procedure. Placement of LARC typically involves a relatively quick bedside procedure; however, the time required to review procedural and device risks and benefits, obtain consent, and answer any remaining questions must be factored into the visit time.

Table 2
How to be reasonably certain that a woman is not pregnant

A health care provider can be reasonably certain that a woman is not pregnant if she has no symptoms or signs of pregnancy and meets any one of the following criteria:

- is ≤7 days after the start of normal menses
- has not had sexual intercourse since the start of last normal menses
- has been correctly and consistently using a reliable method of contraception
- is ≤7 days after spontaneous or induced abortion
- is within 4 weeks postpartum
- is fully or nearly fully breastfeeding (exclusively breastfeeding or the vast majority [≥85%] of feeds are breastfeeds), amenorrheic, and <6 months postpartum

From Curtis KM, Jatlaoui TC, Tepper NK, et al. U.S. Selected Practice Recommendations for Contraceptive Use, 2016. *MMWR Recomm Rep*. 2016;65(4):1-66.

Intrauterine device removals and implant insertions require less time and can be accomplished in a 15- or 20-minute appointment if the consent process is streamlined. In contrast, IUD insertions and implant removals may require additional time to navigate any procedural difficulties that arise and are better suited to a 30-minute appointment. One strategy that may help with patient flow is to reserve LARC procedures for specific days or times of day. While this approach may help with scheduling and time management, it may also limit patient access. To optimize patient access, it is best to allow LARC procedures whenever a credentialed clinician is available (consider same-day insertions), as long as the clinician is reasonably certain the patient is not pregnant and there are no contraindications to placement (Table 2).[7] Practices that are unable to perform same-day insertions should be prepared to offer a short-acting contraceptive method as a temporary bridge until LARC placement. To ensure that patients return for LARC insertion, it is advisable to have a nurse or health educator call or text patients a few days before their procedure to remind them of their appointment and discuss any remaining questions.

Pain Management

It is important to incorporate specific interventions for pain management during IUD and implant placement. It is standard practice to inject 2 mL of 1% lidocaine before implant insertions and removals. Pain management strategies for IUD insertions are more varied. Options for pain management for IUD insertions include analgesics to lessen cramps (prophylactic nonsteroidal anti-inflammatory drugs [NSAIDs]), anesthetics to numb the cervix (paracervical/cervical blocks, topical cervical lidocaine), cervical ripening agents (vaginal or oral misoprostol), and non-pharmacological interventions (music, distraction, preplacement counseling).[8] A recent Cochrane review[9] showed lidocaine 2% gel had no effect on pain during IUD insertion or tenaculum placement. Other forms of lidocaine (topical 4% lidocaine/prilocaine cream, 10% lidocaine spray) showed some effect in nulliparous and parous women. With 1% lidocaine injection, pain at tenaculum placement on the cervix was less compared to no intervention, but there was no difference between the groups in pain with IUD insertion. Those who received misoprostol reported higher pain scores and more cramping than placebo groups. Pain with IUD insertion was less with tramadol versus naproxen; however, in the same trial, pain was less with naproxen compared to placebo.[9]

Ordering and Stocking Supplies

The LARC devices are covered by health insurance plans as either a medical benefit or a pharmacy benefit. When a device is covered as a medical benefit, a practice purchases the device from the manufacturer, designated pharmacy, or specialty distributor and bills the patient's insurance for the device and the procedure.[10] When it is covered as a pharmacy benefit, a pharmacy or specialty distributor bills the insurance carrier directly for the device and the medical provider bills the insurance for the procedure. The medical benefit approach facilitates same-day placements but requires upfront capital (ie, the practice may need to purchase devices and then seek reimbursement after they are placed).[10] The pharmacy benefit reduces the need for upfront capital but may make it difficult for same-day insertions and necessitate delay in insertion appointments. Providers may be eligible for drugs and devices at reduced cost through the 340B drug pricing program, a federal program that requires drug manufacturers to provide outpatient drugs or devices to eligible health care organizations at significantly reduced cost.[10]

Keeping IUDs and implants in stock facilitates same-day insertions and access; however, it may be challenging to estimate patient demand for practices just starting to provide LARC insertion services. The Reproductive Health Supplies Coalition recommends forecasting demand for LARC methods based on patient factors (eg, annual number of females seeking contraception), providers trained to place LARCs, and availability of same-day placement and finance factors.[10] Consider using a fixed monthly ordering system but set a minimum/maximum inventory system.[10]

Medical practices new to providing LARC services should investigate local autoclaving facilities or use affiliated hospital systems for the sterilization of reusable sterile instruments (eg, tenaculum, sound, ring forceps). Tables 3 and 4 list equipment needed for implant and IUD insertions and removals.

Billing and Coding

Correct coding for LARC procedures can result in more appropriate compensation for services. For insertion and removal of LARC methods, report the current procedural terminology (CPT) code that corresponds with the procedure. The CPT codes do not include the cost of the supply. If a practice has supplied

Table 3
Equipment needed for implant insertion and removal

Implant Insertion Supplies	Implant Removal Supplies
Implant insertion and consent forms	Implant removal and consent forms
Povidone-iodine or chlorhexidine swabs	Povidone-iodine or chlorhexidine swabs
2 ml 1% lidocaine with 25-gauge, 1.5-inch needle	2 ml 1% lidocaine with 25-gauge, 0.5-inch or 1.5-inch needle (longer if reinsertion at same time)
Implant package	Scalpel (sterile 15 blade)
Marker	Straight and curved mosquito forceps (sterile)
Gauze 4-inch × 4-inch (sterile)	Gauze 4-inch × 4-inch (sterile)
Alcohol swabs	Alcohol swabs
Adhesive skin closures (Steri-Strips) and pressure bandages	Adhesive skin closures (Steri-Strips) and pressure bandages

Table 4
Equipment needed for IUD insertion and removal

IUD Insertion Supplies	IUD Removal Supplies
IUD insertion procedure and consent forms	IUD removal procedure and consent forms
Water-based lubricant for bimanual examination	Speculum with light source
Speculum with light source	Povidone-iodine or chlorhexidine in cup with cotton-tipped swabs
Sterile gloves	Ring forceps (sterile)
Povidone-iodine or chlorhexidine in cup with large cotton-tipped swabs	Menstrual pad
Ring forceps (sterile)	
Single-toothed tenaculum (sterile)	
Uterine sound (sterile)	
IUD package (open after uterus has been sounded)	
Long suture scissors (sterile)	
Menstrual pad	

IUD, intrauterine device.

the IUD or implant, report the supply separately using the Healthcare Common Procedure Coding System (HCPCS) code.[10] For example, if a practice supplies and places a Kyleena IUD, it would bill the ICD-10 code for Encounter for insertion of an IUD, the CPT code for IUD Insertion, and the HPCS code for Levonorgestrel-releasing IUD, 19.5 mg (Kyleena). If contraceptive counseling or STI screening takes place during the same visit as a LARC procedure, consider reporting an evaluation/management (E/M) service code and the procedure code. If reporting both an E/M service and a procedure, documentation must indicate a significant, separately identifiable E/M service.[10] Consider having a billing and coding specialist review LARC coding to maximize reimbursement.

NAVIGATING CHALLENGES

Although serious complications from LARC placements are rare, pediatricians who plan to provide IUDs and implants should be prepared to address common clinical challenges.

Difficult Placements or Removals

It is not uncommon to encounter difficult IUD placements in young nulliparous adolescents. Consider using a smaller IUD (Kyleena or Skyla), misoprostol, or cervical dilators for young nulliparous adolescents. After a failed IUD insertion refer the patient to a gynecologist, who can place the IUD with ultrasound guidance if necessary. If an implant is not palpable at a follow-up visit, pregnancy should be excluded, and backup contraception provided until the presence of the implant is confirmed; do not attempt removal.[11] The added barium in Nexplanon makes it radiopaque, permitting visualization with 2-dimensional radiography, computerized tomography scan, fluoroscopy, ultrasonography, and magnetic resonance imaging. For non-palpable implants or failed implant removals, refer the patient to an interventional radiologist for removal under ultrasound guidance.[11]

Expulsion and Uterine Perforation

IUD expulsion occurs in 2% to 10% of users and varies by type. Reported risk factors for expulsion include age younger than 20 years, heavy menstrual bleeding, and dysmenorrhea. Uterine perforation occurs once in every 1000 insertions.[11] Most perforations likely occur at the time of insertion and are asymptomatic. Risk factors for expulsion includes less experienced clinicians, postpartum insertions, breastfeeding, and extreme anteflexion/retroflexion of the uterus.[11] Clinicians should visualize IUD strings 4 to 6 weeks after insertion or if the patient presents with irregular bleeding or pain.

Irregular Bleeding and Cramping

Irregular bleeding is expected with both IUDs and implants, as the menstrual cycle is disrupted and ovulation is inhibited. Patients should be counseled on the likelihood of this occurrence before LARC placement. With time, bleeding should become lighter, less painful, and infrequent.[12] If significant irregular bleeding persists 3 to 6 months after placement, consider an underlying gynecologic problem, such as IUD displacement, an STI, or pregnancy. If an underlying problem is not found, consider short-term treatment with NSAIDs or hormonal treatment with oral contraceptives or estrogen.[7] Use of NSAIDs should be encouraged as first-line therapy for dysmenorrhea associated with an IUD.[13] (For additional information on management of bleeding with these devices, see the articles on IUDs by Hoopes and Sucato and contraceptive implants by Gannon-Loew et al in this issue of AM:STARs).

Non-Visualized IUD Strings

String retraction into the cervical canal or uterus is the most common reason for "missing" IUD strings. Uncommonly, non-visualized strings can indicate pregnancy, expulsion, or uterine perforation.[11] An endocervical brush can sometimes be used to retrieve the strings by sweeping the cervical canal. If IUD strings are still not visualized, exclude pregnancy and provide backup contraception until a pelvic ultrasound can be obtained. Once the IUD is visualized in the uterus, no further workup is needed. If an IUD is not seen on ultrasound, obtain an abdominal and pelvic radiograph to evaluate for expulsion or uterine perforation.[11]

Pelvic Inflammatory Disease

Pelvic inflammatory disease (PID) occurs in up to 1% of IUD users despite age or IUD type. The risk of developing PID is highest the first 20 days after IUD insertion.[11] Adolescents should be screened for gonorrhea and chlamydia in advance or at the time of IUD placement. A patient who develops PID may be treated with the IUD left in situ according to Centers for Disease Control and Prevention guidelines. Treatment outcomes are similar whether the IUD is removed or left in place.[11]

SUMMARY

Long-acting reversible contraceptives are ideal options for adolescent and young adult women. Intrauterine devices and implants are the most effective, safe, and economical contraceptive options. Pediatric physicians have a unique opportunity to counsel adolescents and provide them with LARC methods to further reduce teen pregnancy rates. Offering training during residency is the most efficient way to make pediatricians competent in being able to discuss and provide LARC services for their adolescent patients.

QUESTIONS

1. A 16-year-old comes to your office for a follow-up appointment 4 weeks after intrauterine device (IUD) insertion. She complains of heavy bleeding for the past 21 days and is worried. She denies any abdominal cramping

and has not had sex since her IUD was inserted. Her pelvic examination demonstrates visible IUD strings at the cervix. What is the most appropriate next step in management?
A. Send for pelvic ultrasound.
B. Recommend IUD removal given heavy bleeding.
C. Discuss a trial of oral contraceptives for 1 month.
D. Discuss a trial of scheduled acetaminophen for 1 week.

2. A 17-year-old nulliparous female presents for IUD placement. She is worried about the pain of insertion. Which of the following measures to alleviate the pain of an IUD insertion is supported by evidence from clinical trials?
A. Recommend she take misoprostol before placement.
B. Use 2% lidocaine gel before inserting the IUD.
C. Provide prophylactic naproxen.
D. Administer an anxiolytic.

3. A 15-year-old female presents for implant follow-up. She denies any concerns with the method and reports her cycles have lightened. On examination, you are unable to palpate the implant in her left upper arm. What is the next appropriate step in management?
A. Advise her to return in 2 weeks for repeat examination.
B. Check for pregnancy and provide a backup method.
C. Obtain a computerized tomography scan.
D. Send her to interventional radiology for removal.

(See page 203 for answers.)

References

1. Committee on Practice Bulletin-Gynecology, Long-Acting Reversible Conception Work Group. Practice Bulletin No. 186: Long-acting reversible conception: implants and intrauterine devices. *Obstet Gynecol.* 2017;130(5):e251-e269
2. Smith AJB, Harney KF, Singh T, Hurwitz AG. Provider and health system factors associated with usage of long-acting reversible contraception in adolescents. *J Pediatr Adolesc Gynecol.* 2017;30:609-614
3. Potter J, Koyama A, Coles MS. Addressing the challenges of clinician training for long-acting reversible contraception. *JAMA Pediatr.* 2015;169(2):103-104
4. American Academy of Pediatrics Committee on Adolescence. Contraception for adolescents. *Pediatrics.* 2014;134(4):e1244-e1256
5. ACOG Committee Opinion No. 735: Adolescents and long-acting reversible contraception: implants and intrauterine devices. *Obstet Gynecol.* 2018;131(5):e130-e139
6. Eisenberg D, McNicholas C, Peripert JE. Cost as a barrier to long-acting reversible contraceptive (LARC) use in adolescents. *J Adolesc Health.* 2013;52(4 Suppl):S59-S63
7. Curtis KM, Jatlaoui TC, Tepper NK, et al. U.S. Selected Practice Recommendations for Contraceptive Use, 2016. *MMWR Recomm Rep.* 2016;65(4):1-66
8. Francis JK, Gold MA. Long-acting reversible contraception for adolescents: a review. *JAMA Pediatr.* 2017;171(7):694-701

9. Lopez LM, Bernholc A, Zeng Y, et al. Interventions for pain with intrauterine device insertion (review). *Cochrane Database Syst Rev.* 2015;7:CD007373
10. Armstrong E, McKee C, Gandal-Powers M, et al. Intrauterine devices and implants: a guide to reimbursement. http://larcprogram.ucsf.edu. Updated April 6, 2016. Accessed June 13, 2018
11. American College of Obstetricians and Gynecologists' Committee on Gynecologic Practice, Long-Acting Reversible Contraception Expert Working Group. Committee Opinion No. 672: clinical challenges of long-acting reversible contraceptive methods. *Obstet Gynecol.* 2016;128(3):e69-e77
12. Allen S, Barlow E. Long-acting reversible contraception: an essential guide for pediatric primary care providers. *Pediatr Clin N Am.* 2017;64:359-369
13. Hillard PJ. Practical tips for intrauterine devices use in adolescents. *J Adolesc Health.* 2013; 52(4 Suppl):S40-S46

Adolesc Med 030 (2019) 161–173

Special Cases: Case-Based Contraception Scenarios

Sofya Maslyanskaya, MD[a]; Susan M. Coupey, MD[b*]

[a]Assistant Professor of Pediatrics, Division of Adolescent Medicine, Children's Hospital at Montefiore, Albert Einstein College of Medicine, Bronx, New York; [b]Professor of Pediatrics, Chief Emerita, Division of Adolescent Medicine, Children's Hospital at Montefiore, Albert Einstein College of Medicine, Bronx, New York

LEARNING OBJECTIVES

After reviewing this article, the reader should be able to:

1. Describe the management steps for patients after their contraceptive implant or intrauterine device (IUD) is not located in the expected position on examination
2. Describe the management of a young woman with a malpositioned IUD
3. List the non-contraceptive benefits of hormonal contraceptives for adolescents with bleeding disorders and intellectual disabilities

INTRODUCTION

Long-acting reversible contraceptive use by adolescents has increased in the past decade. Awareness of complications and common problems encountered with subdermal contraceptive implant and intrauterine device (IUD) use is essential for provision of optimal contraceptive management for adolescent patients. The provision of levonorgestrel IUDs for medically complex patients may assist with both contraceptive management and treatment of their medical conditions.

*Corresponding author
E-mail address: scoupey@montefiore.org

 ISSN 1934-4287

CASE 1: NON-PALPABLE CONTRACEPTIVE IMPLANT

A 17-year-old girl who had her contraceptive implant inserted into her left upper arm 3 years ago comes in for implant removal and reinsertion because of expiration of the current device. During the physical examination, before starting the removal procedure, you are unable to palpate the implant in her left arm.

The use of subdermal contraceptive implants by adolescents in the United States (US) has been increasing over the last decade. The National Survey of Family Growth (NSFG) found that between 2011 and 2015, the implant was used by 3% of teenagers aged 15 to19 years compared to 1% between 2006 and 2010.[1] The current implant available in the United States is Nexplanon, which is a 4-cm, rod-shaped device containing 68 mg of the progestin hormone etonogestrel. Contraceptive implants are among the most effective types of contraception available.[2-4] They are easily inserted and do not involve invasive gynecologic procedures such as pelvic examinations. Implants have been found to be a highly acceptable form of hormonal contraception in teenagers. In the Contraceptive CHOICE Project cohort, a prospective study that aimed to increase use of effective contraception by providing devices and medications at no cost, 50% of 14- to-17-year-old girls selected the implant compared to 26% of 18- and 19-year-old women.[5] As the rate of implant use increases, pediatricians and other clinicians (eg, family medicine physicians, gynecologists, physician assistants, and nurse practitioners, collectively referred to as *clinicians*) caring for adolescents need to be aware of the rare possibility of implant migration and the need to assess for implant location.

Subdermal contraceptive implants are inserted into the inner side of the upper arm 8 to 10 cm from the medial epicondyle of the humerus, taking special care to prevent insertion of the implant into the medial bicipital groove between the biceps and triceps. A letter reviewing this technique was sent to US health care practitioners in the fall of 2015 by Merck & Co., the makers of Nexplanon, after findings of migration to distant sites were reported in the postmarketing adverse events data.[6] Before insertion, the clinician should assess for the presence of the implant in the inserter device. After insertion but before bandage application, both the clinician and the patient should feel for the device under the skin to ensure its presence. The patient is instructed to intermittently check for implant location and return for reevaluation if she is unable to palpate it.

Inability to palpate an implant at the time of removal is rare.[7] If this occurs, the clinician should assess the location of the implant using a stepwise method. Nexplanon, the only implant currently available in the United States, differs from its predecessor Implanon by having an improved inserter device and the addition of barium sulfate, which makes it radiopaque. If the implant is not palpable on physical examination, the first step in the investigation before proceeding any further is to obtain a radiograph of the arm in which the implant was inserted. If the implant is not visualized on the radiograph, the next step is to obtain a chest radiograph. If the adolescent has an Implanon that is not radiopaque, then the imaging modality should be either an ultrasound or magnetic resonance scan of the arm and chest.

The standard procedure for implant removal includes palpation of the device, marking of the removal site (which should be at the distal tip of the implant), cleansing of the injection site, administration of local anesthesia, and creation of a 2 mm incision at the distal tip of the implant. The implant is removed by grasping the distal end with forceps while pushing the proximal edge toward the incision site. Outpatient office procedures should not involve any deep dissection. Removal of an implant should never be attempted if the implant is not palpable. If imaging is required to locate the implant, then removal should proceed under ultrasound guidance or in the operating room.

A study of the US Food and Drug Administration Adverse Event Reporting System database in 2017 revealed only 38 cases of distant implant migration.[8] Of the 38 cases, 9 implants had migrated to the lung/pulmonary artery, 14 to vasculature other than the lung/pulmonary artery, and 15 to extravascular sites such as axilla, clavicle, neck, and chest wall. Most cases originated in the United States and France. Few patients presented with symptoms of shortness of breath and discomfort, and most cases were discovered only when the patient requested implant removal. In this cohort, 16 patients required surgical removal in an operating room, including 1 requiring lung segmentectomy and 1 thoracotomy. Based on the results of this study, implant migration to the pulmonary artery is likely to occur in less than 1 in 7000 insertions. Merck and Co. estimates that migration to vasculature occurs in 1.3 per one million of devices sold.[9] This is based on data recorded in the global safety databases between August 1998 and April 2015. Multiple case reports of implants migrating to pulmonary vasculature have been described.[10,11] One reported axillary migration of the implant occurred in a patient with spastic cerebral palsy.[12]

A systematic review of the literature performed in 2017 described the types of nerve injuries sustained during implant insertions and removals.[12] The study found 12 patients, with one-third each having complications secondary to Norplant (an implant that has been removed from the market), Implanon, and Nexplanon use. In 7 patients the implants were not palpable, and in 1 patient palpation was not documented before attempted implant removal. The neurologic findings included paresthesias in 11 patients, weakness in 6 patients, and loss of sensation in 8 patients. Most of the nerve injuries occurred at the time of device removal, and the nerves most commonly injured were the median nerve and the medial antebrachial cutaneous nerve. The injuries occurred during implant removal when the clinician mistook the nerve for the implant and pulled on the nerve.

A possible contributor to migration seems to be improper and deep placement during implant insertion. The associations between patient and physician characteristics and difficult implant removals were studied in adult women presenting to a hospital-based gynecologic practice in France.[13] When comparing standard to difficult implant removals, the study found that weight gain of more than 1 kg, insertion performed in a private practice, and duration of implant use (>25 months) were all independently associated with a higher likelihood of difficult removal. Based on these results, the study recommended that additional training and supervision of new clinicians be standard to prevent deep or improper insertion techniques.

Implants are safe and effective forms of contraception for adolescents. Nonpalpable implants are rare events that should be evaluated by locating the implant with imaging techniques. Based on the location and anatomic involvement, a surgical or interventional radiology consultation may be necessary for implant removal with ultrasound or computed tomography guidance. It may also need to be performed in the operating room to prevent further complications such as neurovascular injury. Supervision of junior clinicians is advised to prevent incorrect insertion techniques.

CASE 2: MISSING IUD STRINGS

A 21-year-old woman comes in for routine gynecologic care. She is being transitioned to adult care after this visit and is due for her first Pap smear. She had an IUD inserted 2 years ago for contraceptive management. After an external genital examination, you insert a speculum and do not visualize her IUD strings.

Based on the National Survey of Family Growth, IUDs were used by 3% of 15- to 19-year-old adolescents between 2011 and 2015.[1] Currently on the market in the United States are multiple hormonal IUDs, which all contain varying amounts of the progestin levonorgestrel, and 1 non-hormonal copper IUD. They are safe, effective methods of contraception and have high levels of satisfaction among adolescents.[14,15]

The inability to visualize IUD stings on inspection of the cervix is a relatively common issue, occurring in up to 16% of patients.[16] A comprehensive history, including menstrual history before and after IUD insertion, current menstrual bleeding pattern, and whether the IUD strings were previously palpated by the patient or visualized by a clinician should help with the differential diagnosis of missing IUD strings. More than one-third of women with levonorgestrel IUDs experience amenorrhea.[17,18] Women with copper IUDs have heavier and more painful menses than before insertion of the device.[19] Thus, a recent change in bleeding pattern to either heavier or lighter bleeding depending on the type of IUD inserted may signal expulsion of the device.

The differential diagnosis of missing IUD strings includes an unnoticed expulsion, presence of the IUD in the abdominal cavity after perforation of the uterus, rotation of the IUD such that the strings were retracted into the cervical canal or uterus, or broken strings. Retraction of the IUD strings is the most common reason for absent strings on examination. In a review of almost 1500 charts of women with IUDs, 5% of the patients had absent strings on examination. Of these 5% of women with absent strings, 98% of the IUDs were visualized in the uterine cavity on ultrasound, just over 1% had been expelled, and less than 1% were found in the pelvis.[20]

Expulsions occur in up to 10% of IUD users, with teenagers 14 to 19 years old and parous women more likely to experience expulsions.[21,22] If the adolescent in this case had expelled her levonorgestrel IUD and was previously amenorrheic, then she should have noticed a change in her menstrual cycle pattern with return of menses or dysmenorrhea. For adolescents with a copper IUD, an expulsion may be noted by a change to lighter and less painful menses or amenorrhea secondary to pregnancy. A pregnancy test is indicated when IUD strings are not visible.

Uterine perforations during IUD insertions are rare, occurring at a rate of about 0.1%.[23,24] Perforations are usually noted at the time of IUD insertion, with pain, bleeding, and missing strings noted after IUD placement. Infrequently the patient is asymptomatic, and the perforation is noted at the time of IUD removal. In a study of a surgical database, 43% of the 37 women with a surgical diagnosis of uterine perforation over a 14-year time period had no symptoms at the time of diagnosis.[25] If a uterine perforation had occurred at the time of a levonorgestrel IUD insertion, the patient may still become amenorrheic secondary to systemic release of the levonorgestrel hormone.

During a standard IUD removal procedure, the clinician visualizes the strings protruding from the external cervical os, grasps the strings using forceps, and pulls gently with or without use of traction on the cervix with a tenaculum. If the clinician is not able to visualize the IUD strings, the first step should be an attempt to sweep the strings into view by using a cervical cytology brush. If the patient is amenorrheic and the strings are not visualized, then a pregnancy test should be performed. In addition, the adolescent should be advised to abstain from sexual activity or use backup contraception until ultrasound is performed to assess for location of the IUD. For patients in whom the IUD is not visualized in the uterus on ultrasound, a radiograph of the pelvis and abdomen should be performed to assess for the location of the IUD device. This radiograph should assess the upper abdominal quadrants and the dependent portion of the pelvis. This is important, as locating the IUD in the pelvic or abdominal cavity with indication of a uterine perforation would require prompt removal of the IUD in the operating room.

Removal of an intrauterine IUD with missing strings can be performed safely as an office procedure under ultrasound guidance, thus eliminating the need for anesthesia and the additional cost associated with an operating room procedure. In a study of 23 women presenting for ultrasound-guided IUD removal, 83% were successfully removed during office procedures; the rest required hysteroscopic removal.[26] Clinicians have a choice of forceps with varying degrees of opening length from the joint of the device. Patterson alligator forceps have a short opening length that allows the instrument to open fully within the uterine cavity to easily grasp the device or the strings. Polyp forceps have a long opening length, and the ability to maneuver them within the uterine cavity and grasp the device or the strings may be limited.[27] During an intrauterine IUD removal, the patient should be made comfortable by providing analgesia and possibly cervical dilation. Cervical dilation can be achieved using an osmotic dilator (eg, Lamicel), a synthetic hydrophilic polymer, or a laminaria tent made from stems of algae (*Laminaria japomica* or *Laminaria digitate)*. Both of these require insertion by a clinician into the cervical canal.[14,15] Another option is intravaginal placement of misoprostol, a prostaglandin analogue, several hours before the procedure. Analgesia can be achieved with a paracervical block or with conscious sedation.

While missing IUD strings at the time of pelvic examinations are relatively common, uterine perforations are rare. Standard office procedures as described above should be implemented to locate the missing IUD strings. Next steps in providing ongoing reproductive health care for the patient should be based on the location of the IUD.

CASE 3: MALPOSITIONED IUD

An 18-year-old woman who had a levonorgestrel IUD inserted 2 years ago comes in for a follow-up visit. She reports that she has recently experienced pelvic cramps several times a month and relates it to her IUD. On pelvic examination, you visualize the strings, and transvaginal ultrasound reveals the IUD stem partially located in the cervical canal.

The standard IUD position in the uterus is at the top of the fundus with the arms parallel to the fundus and perpendicular to the stem in a T shape. Malpositioned IUDs may be found anywhere, from a few centimeters below the fundus to partially or completely positioned within the cervical canal (rotated or embedded into the myometrium). Currently, because of limited evidence for the appropriate approach to a malpositioned IUD, clinicians make decisions on a case-by-case basis. A study of senior physicians in United Kingdom and Australia found that 80% would remove and replace both copper and levonorgestrel IUDs if they were lying partially or completely in the cervical canal.[28]

There are several studies of contraceptive effectiveness of malpositioned IUDs that can help to guide clinicians' decisions about the approach. One 6-year observational study of women with copper IUDs followed for routine care looked at IUD positioning in 318 women with copper IUDs who became pregnant compared to 300 women with copper IUDs who did not become pregnant. The study found that 64% of the pregnant women had a malpositioned IUD compared to only 11% of the non-pregnant women.[29] A 2005 study evaluating the use of a novel, differently shaped IUD device containing 52 mg of levonorgestrel randomly assigned 298 women to intrauterine (fundal) or cervical canal insertions and found that the rate of pregnancy and expulsion, pain, or bleeding did not differ by insertion location.[30] These 2 studies suggest that malposition of the device may be associated with lower contraceptive efficacy for the copper IUD but not for the levonorgestrel IUD. However, when making the decision on whether to remove a malpositioned IUD, adverse effects such as bleeding and pain should be taken into consideration. A retrospective case control study of women with malpositioned IUDs that were removed compared to women with IUDs in the normal uterine fundal position found a higher rate of pregnancy in the women with malpositioned IUDs and showed the importance of providing alternative contraception at the time of removal of a malpositioned IUD.[31]

The necessity of a follow-up appointment after IUD insertion and the appropriate timing of that appointment were evaluated in multiple studies. A systematic review found 4 studies that assessed frequency of follow-up and found that neither removal of an IUD for medical reasons nor longer duration of IUD use occurred in women who had more frequent follow-up appointments.[32] Therefore, the US Selected Practice Recommendations for Contraceptive Use published by the Centers for Disease Control and Prevention advise that no routine follow-up visit should be required but recommend that physicians consider IUD string checks at other visits following the insertion and consider frequent visits for adolescent patients.[33] Patients who present with abnormal uterine bleeding or pain are more likely than those without symptoms to have a malpositioned IUD detected by ultrasonography when a 3-dimensional coronal view of the uterus is used.[34]

In women with IUDs, symptoms of new pelvic pain or unexpected change in menstrual pattern should prompt an evaluation for IUD location. The clinician's approach to partially expelled IUDs should be made on a case by case basis.

CASE 4: GIRL WITH MENORRHAGIA AND VON WILLEBRAND FACTOR DEFICIENCY NEEDING CONTRACEPTION

A 16-year-old girl comes to you for contraceptive management. She reports that she has experienced prolonged uterine bleeding since menarche, with menses occurring monthly and lasting for 2 weeks. On screening evaluation, she has a low level of von Willebrand factor.

Von Willebrand disease (vWD) occurs in up 1% of the general population.[35-37] Up to one-third of women with heavy or prolonged menstrual bleeding are found to have vWD.[38-40] For the adolescent with vWD who is sexually active, the levonorgestrel IUD is the best option because of its high efficacy for both contraception and cessation of heavy menses.[41-43] Levonorgestrel IUDs have been found to increase median hemoglobin concentrations and quality-of-life scores.[44] In studies of women with vWD, almost half became amenorrheic after levonorgestrel IUD insertion; the remainder had markedly fewer bleeding days than before IUD insertion. A study of adolescents with bleeding disorders who had a levonorgestrel IUD inserted under anesthesia and had periprocedural treatment with desmopressin and/or antifibrinolytic therapy found that the adolescents had improvement in symptoms within 1 to 5 months after insertion, with 60% achieving amenorrhea.[44] A systematic review of hormonal contraception as a treatment of abnormal uterine bleeding found that compared to combined oral contraceptive (COC) pills and depot medroxyprogesterone acetate (DMPA), levonorgestrel IUDs were more effective at reducing menstrual blood loss.[45] Use of subdermal contraceptive implants has not been studied for treatment of heavy menstrual bleeding but are more likely than levonorgestrel IUDs to cause intermenstrual bleeding. The COC pills may work by increasing levels of factor VIII and von Willebrand factor, whereas DMPA and levonorgestrel IUDs work by decreasing the thickness of the endometrium. In addition, levonorgestrel IUDs may be associated with decreased flow in uterine spiral arteries.[46] Other medications that may be used in conjunction with the levonorgestrel IUD or COC pills to control menstrual bleeding include desmopressin and antifibrinolytics such as tranexamic acid.

Girls and women with vWD frequently experience heavy and prolonged uterine bleeding. Hormonal contraceptives, in particular the levonorgestrel IUD, can provide excellent bleeding control, prevent iron-deficiency anemia and have the additional benefit of providing effective contraception for the young women who need it.

CASE 5: GIRL WITH MODERATE INTELLECTUAL DISABILITY AND BEHAVIORAL CHANGES WITH MENSES NEEDING CONTRACEPTION

A 17-year-old girl with moderate intellectual disability is brought in by her mother for evaluation of behavioral changes with menses. The mother also reports that she has noticed that her daughter has a male friend whom she hugs and holds hands with, and the mother is worried about potential sexual activity and pregnancy.

Menstrual management can be challenging for parents of girls with intellectual disabilities. For girls with both intellectual and physical disabilities, menstruation can create an increased burden on caregivers for hygiene and may be associated with behavioral changes related to physical changes (eg, menorrhagia, dysmenorrhea, and increased seizure frequency).

Several different types of hormonal suppression (COCs, DMPA, levonorgestrel IUD, and implants) may be offered based on reported symptoms and the end result desired by the family.

In the past, DMPA was the most commonly selected method for adolescents with intellectual and physical disabilities because it provides menstrual suppression and often causes amenorrhea by profoundly suppressing the hypothalamic-pituitary-ovarian axis. Its use has recently declined because of concern for impaired bone mineral accrual and low bone density related to hypoestrogenemia. One study of Canadian adolescents with intellectual and physical disabilities reviewed the records of menstrual suppression for 72 patients from 1998 to 2003 compared with 300 patients from 2006 to 2011. The study found that DMPA use declined from 58% to 12%, with an increase in extended use of COC pills from 17% to 42%.[47] The study also found that in the 2006 to 2011 cohort, the hormonal contraceptive patch was used in 20% of the patients and the levonorgestrel IUD in 3%.

The risks, benefits, and alternatives need to be weighed when hormonal contraceptives are used for menstrual suppression. Continuous COC pills have a possible risk of deep venous thrombosis, and intravaginal rings pose an additional concern for girls who are not able to insert the ring themselves as they would need to undergo monthly intravaginal insertions by a parent or guardian. Levonorgestrel IUDs are used for treatment of women with menorrhagia and have recently begun being used for girls with intellectual and physical disabilities. Most of these girls require IUD insertion under sedation, which is an additional risk. In a study of 21 adolescent girls with developmental delay, 20 required general anesthesia for the gynecologic examination and IUD insertion.[48] Continuation of IUD use by the adolescents in this study was high, with only 1 request for removal after 11 months. Many children's hospitals provide a conscious sedation service for children requiring brief painful same-day procedures, such as a renal biopsy, and this service can be used for IUD insertion in adolescents with intellectual and physical disabilities, with less risk than general anesthesia.

In summary, multiple hormonal options are available that may be used for contraception as well as menstrual suppression in girls with intellectual and physical disabilities. The options should be reviewed with the family and the adolescent, if possible, and the decision on the method type should be made jointly between the family and the clinician. Education and guidance on the anticipated decrease in menstrual blood flow should occur at the time of counseling.

QUESTIONS

1. A 17-year-old girl comes to your office for removal of her subdermal contraceptive implant (Nexplanon). You are not able to palpate the implant in her left arm at the site of insertion. What is the best next step?
   A. Ultrasound of the left upper arm
   B. Radiograph of the left upper arm
   C. Attempt to remove the implant by making an incision at the site of insertion
   D. Magnetic resonance imaging of the chest
2. An 18-year-old woman who had a levonorgestrel intrauterine device (IUD) inserted 2 years ago and had become amenorrheic after the insertion reports that she started menstruating monthly 3 months ago and had her last menstrual period 3 weeks ago. What is the next best step in assessing the reason for her monthly menses?
   A. Urine pregnancy test
   B. Urine chlamydia and gonorrhea nucleic acid amplification testing
   C. Gynecologic examination with cervical inspection for IUD strings
   D. Pelvic ultrasound
3. A 16-year-old girl with type 1 von Willebrand disease and low von Willebrand factor level is seen for evaluation of menstrual bleeding after a trial of tranexamic acid for treatment of menorrhagia. During the private interview time, she reports that she is sexually active and has a male partner. What method(s) should you recommend for treatment of menorrhagia and contraceptive management?
   A. Combined hormonal contraceptive pills
   B. Levonorgestrel IUD
   C. Subdermal contraceptive implant
   D. Copper IUD
   E. A and B only
   F. B and D only

(See pages 203-204 for answers.)

References

1. Abma JC, Martinez G. Sexual activity and contraceptive use among teenagers in the United States, 2011-2015. *Natl Health Stat Rep.* 2017;104:1-23
2. McNicholas C, Maddipati R, Zhao Q, Swor E, Peipert JF. Use of the etonogestrel implant and levonorgestrel intrauterine device beyond the US Food and Drug Administration–approved duration. *Obstetrics and gynecology.* 2015;125(3):599-604
3. Croxatto HB, Urbancsek J, Massai R, Bennink HC, van Beek A. A multicentre efficacy and safety study of the single contraceptive implant Implanon®. *Human Reproduction.* 1999;14(4):976-981
4. Ali M, Akin A, Bahamondes L, et al. Extended use up to 5 years of the etonogestrel-releasing subdermal contraceptive implant: comparison to levonorgestrel-releasing subdermal implant. *Human Reproduction.* 2016;31(11):2491-2498
5. Secura GM, Madden T, McNicholas C, et al. Provision of no-cost, long-acting contraception and teenage pregnancy. *N Engl J Med.* 2014;371(14):1316-1323
6. Nexplanon-etonogestrel implant. US Food and Drug Administration (FDA) approved product information. Revised May 2017. US National Library of Medicine. www.dailymed.nlm.nih.gov https://dailymed.nlm.nih.gov/dailymed/drugInfo.cfm?setid=b03a3917-9a65-45c2-bbbb-871da858ef34. Accessed on October 24, 2016
7. Darney P, Patel A, Rosen K, Shapiro LS, Kaunitz AM. Safety and efficacy of a single-rod etonogestrel implant (Implanon): results from 11 international clinical trials. *Fertil Steril.* 2009;91(5): 1646-1653
8. Kang S, Niak A, Gada N, Brinker A, Jones SC. Etonogestrel implant migration to the vasculature, chest wall, and distant body sites: cases from a pharmacovigilance database. *Contraception.* 2017;96(6):439-445
9. MSD. Nexplanon (etonogestrel): implants have been found rarely in the vasculature and lung. An update regarding possible risks and complications regarding insertion, localization and removal. https://assets.publishing.service.gov.uk/media/576006d640f0b652dd000036/Nexplanon_DHPC_sent_31_May_2016.pdf. Published May 31, 2016. Accessed November 26, 2018
10. Gao GT, Binder W. Embolization of a contraceptive implant into the pulmonary vasculature in an adolescent female. *Am J Emerg Med.* 2018;36(6):1122.e1-1122.e2
11. Barlow-Evans R, Jaffer K, Balogun M. Migration of a Nexplanon contraceptive implant to the pulmonary artery. *BMJ Case Reports.* 2017;pii: bcr-2017-219259
12. Laumonerie P, Blasco L, Tibbo ME, et al. Peripheral nerve injury associated with a subdermal contraceptive implant: illustrative cases and systematic review of literature. *World Neurosurg.* 2018;111:317-325
13. Chevreau J, Krief D, Arab OA, et al. Factors associated with removal difficulties of etonogestrel-containing contraceptive implants (Nexplanon®). *Eur J Obstet Gynecol Reprod Biol.* 2018;224: 81-84
14. Peipert JF, Zhao Q, Allsworth JE, et al. Continuation and satisfaction of reversible contraception. *Obstet Gynecol.* 2011;117(5):1105-1113
15. Friedman JO. Factors associated with contraceptive satisfaction in adolescent women using the IUD. *J Pediatr Adolesc Gynecol.* 2015;28(1):38-42
16. Tugrul S, Yavuzer B, Yildirim G, Kayahan A. The duration of use, causes of discontinuation, and problems during removal in women admitted for removal of IUD. *Contraception.* 2005;71(2): 149-152
17. Hidalgo M, Bahamondes L, Perrotti M, Diaz J, Dantas-Monteiro C, Petta C. Bleeding patterns and clinical performance of the levonorgestrel-releasing intrauterine system (Mirena) up to two years. *Contraception.* 2002;65(2):129-132

18. Carvalho NM, Chou V, Modesto W, Margatho D, Garcia EAL, Bahamondes L. Relationship between user satisfaction with the levonorgestrel-releasing intrauterine system and bleeding patterns. *J Obstet Gynaecol Res.* 2017;43(11):1732-1737
19. Kaneshiro B, Aeby T. Long-term safety, efficacy, and patient acceptability of the intrauterine Copper T-380A contraceptive device. *Int J Womens Health.* 2010;2:211-220
20. Marchi NM, Castro S, Hidalgo MM, et al. Management of missing strings in users of intrauterine contraceptives. *Contraception.* 2012;86(4):354-358
21. Madden T, McNicholas C, Zhao Q, Secura GM, Eisenberg DL, Peipert JF. Association of age and parity with intrauterine device expulsion. *Obstet Gynecol.* 2014;124(4):718-726
22. Sivin I, El Mahgoub S, McCarthy T, et al. Long-term contraception with the levonorgestrel 20 mcg/day (LNg 20) and the copper T 380Ag intrauterine devices: a five-year randomized study. *Contraception.* 1990;42(4):361-378
23. Chi I, Feldblum P, Rogers S. IUD-related uterine perforation: an epidemiologic analysis of a rare event using an international dataset. *Contracept Deliv Syst.* 1984;5(2):123-130
24. Heinemann K, Reed S, Moehner S, Do Minh T. Risk of uterine perforation with levonorgestrel-releasing and copper intrauterine devices in the European Active Surveillance Study on Intrauterine Devices. *Contraception.* 2015;91(4):274-279
25. Kho KA, Chamsy DJ. Perforated intraperitoneal intrauterine contraceptive devices: diagnosis, management, and clinical outcomes. *J Minim Invasive Gynecol.* 2014;21(4):596-601
26. Verma U, Astudillo-Dávalos FE, Gerkowicz SA. Safe and cost-effective ultrasound guided removal of retained intrauterine device: our experience. *Contraception.* 2015;92(1):77-80
27. Prabhakaran S, Chuang A. In-office retrieval of intrauterine contraceptive devices with missing strings. *Contraception.* 2011;83(2):102-106
28. Golightly E, Gebbie AE. Clinicians' views on low-lying intrauterine devices or systems. *J Fam Plann Reprod Health Care.* 2014;40(2):113-116
29. İnal MM, Ertopçu K, Özelmas İ. The evaluation of 318 intrauterine pregnancy cases with an intrauterine device. *Eur J Contracept Reprod Health Care.* 2005;10(4):266-271
30. Pakarinen P, Luukkainen T. Five years' experience with a small intracervical/intrauterine levonorgestrel-releasing device. *Contraception.* 2005;72(5):342-345
31. Braaten KP, Benson CB, Maurer R, Goldberg AB. Malpositioned intrauterine contraceptive devices: risk factors, outcomes, and future pregnancies. *Obstet Gynecol.* 2011;118(5):1014-1020
32. Steenland MW, Zapata LB, Brahmi D, Marchbanks PA, Curtis KM. The effect of follow-up visits or contacts after contraceptive initiation on method continuation and correct use. *Contraception.* 2013;87(5):625-630
33. Curtis KM, Jatlaoui TC, Tepper NK, et al. U.S. selected practice recommendations for contraceptive use, 2016. *MMWR Recomm Rep.* 2016;65(4):1-66
34. Benacerraf B, Shipp T, Bromley B. Three-dimensional ultrasound detection of abnormally located intrauterine contraceptive devices which are a source of pelvic pain and abnormal bleeding. *Ultrasound Obstet Gynecol.* 2009;34(1):110-115
35. Rodeghiero F, Castaman G, Dini E. Epidemiological investigation of the prevalence of von Willebrand's disease. *Blood.* 1987;69(2):454-459
36. Bowman M, Hopman W, Rapson D, Lillicrap D, James P. The prevalence of symptomatic von Willebrand disease in primary care practice. *J Thromb Haemost.* 2010;8(1):213-216
37. Werner EJ, Broxson EH, Tucker EL, Giroux DS, Shults J, Abshire TC. Prevalence of von Willebrand disease in children: a multiethnic study. *J Pediatr.* 1993;123(6):893-898
38. Rodriguez V, Alme C, Killian JM, Weaver AL, Khan SP, Simmons PS. Bleeding disorders in adolescents with menorrhagia: an institutional experience. *Haemophilia.* 2013;19(2):e101-e102
39. Diaz R, Dietrich JE, Mahoney D Jr, Yee DL, Srivaths LV. Hemostatic abnormalities in young females with heavy menstrual bleeding. *J Pediatr Adolesc Gynecol.* 2014;27(6):324-329
40. Mikhail S, Varadarajan R, Kouides P. The prevalence of disorders of haemostasis in adolescents with menorrhagia referred to a haemophilia treatment centre. *Haemophilia.* 2007;13(5):627-632

41. Heinemann K, Reed S, Moehner S, Do Minh T. Comparative contraceptive effectiveness of levonorgestrel-releasing and copper intrauterine devices: the European Active Surveillance Study for Intrauterine Devices. *Contraception.* 2015;91(4):280-283
42. Winner B, Peipert JF, Zhao Q, et al. Effectiveness of long-acting reversible contraception. *N Engl J Med.* 2012;366(21):1998-2007
43. Stewart A, Cummins C, Gold L, Jordan R, Phillips W. The effectiveness of the levonorgestrel-releasing intrauterine system in menorrhagia: a systematic review. *BJOG.* 2001;108(1):74-86
44. Adeyemi-Fowode OA, Santos XM, Dietrich JE, Srivaths L. Levonorgestrel-releasing intrauterine device use in female adolescents with heavy menstrual bleeding and bleeding disorders: single institution review. *J Pediatr Adolesc Gynecol.* 2017;30(4):479-483
45. Uhm S, Perriera L. Hormonal contraception as treatment for heavy menstrual bleeding: a systematic review. *Clin Obstet Gynecol.* 2014;57(4):694-717
46. Bastianelli C, Farris M, Rapiti S, Bruno Vecchio R, Benagiano G. Different bleeding patterns with the use of levonorgestrel intrauterine system: are they associated with changes in uterine artery blood flow? *Biomed Res Int.* 2014;2014:815127
47. Kirkham YA, Allen L, Kives S, Caccia N, Spitzer RF, Ornstein MP. Trends in menstrual concerns and suppression in adolescents with developmental disabilities. *J Adolesc Health.* 2013;53(3):407-412
48. Hillard PJ. Menstrual suppression with the levonorgestrel intrauterine system in girls with developmental delay. *J Pediatr Adolesc Gynecol.* 2012;25(5):308-313

Adolesc Med 030 (2019) 174–186

Policy Foundations Supporting Adolescent Access to Contraceptive Care

Laura K. Grubb, MD, MPH[a*];
Krishna K. Upadhya, MD, MPH[b]

[a]*Director, Adolescent Medicine, Assistant Professor of Pediatrics, Assistant Professor of Public Health and Community Medicine, Floating Hospital for Children at Tufts Medical Center, Boston, Massachusetts;*
[b]*Assistant Professor, Division of Adolescent and Young Adult Medicine, Children's National Health System, Washington, DC*

LEARNING OBJECTIVES

After reviewing this article, the reader should be able to:

1. Discuss broad principles of policies that affect access to contraception, including consent, confidentiality, payment issues, availability of contraception, and conscientious objection
2. Discuss trends in policies affecting contraception access and availability, ongoing changes, and possible future directions
3. Provide resources for health care clinicians to access information on contraception access and availability, including sites that track changes and provide avenues for advocacy

INTRODUCTION

Adolescents' access to contraception and contraceptive services is vital to healthy sexuality, health promotion, prevention of unintended pregnancies, and treatment of common adolescent gynecologic problems. Adolescents face unique challenges to contraceptive access, including issues of consent, confidentiality (of both services and insurance), cost, and conscientious objection. These challenges have significant effects on adolescent health and quality of life.

*Corresponding author
E-mail address: LGrubb@tuftsmedicalcenter.org

 ISSN 1934-4287

MINORS' CONSENT FOR CONTRACEPTION

Before rendering any health service, health care clinicians must consider the patient's right and ability to consent to receive that service. In the case of minors, the right to consent for health care is not absolute. In fact, for most health care services, the right of minors is limited, and parents or legal guardians must provide consent. Contraception, and other health services for which minors may desire a high degree of privacy, are often exceptions, with federal or state statutes allowing minors to consent on their own to encourage the use of services that may otherwise be foregone.

Many institutions and organizations support the rights of the adolescent to consent for contraception services. In 1994, the United Nations globally recognized minor adolescents' rights to contraception information and services.[1] The 2015 American Public Health Association (APHA) policy statement Universal Access to Contraception iterated, "APHA strongly urges protection and fulfillment of universal rights to safe, voluntary, confidential access to the full range of contraceptive methods without barriers, regardless of age, marital status, gender identity, ethnicity, sexual orientation, religious background, socioeconomic status, geography, health status (including chronic disease, especially HIV/AIDS), nationality, or other demographic characteristics."[2] Specifically with regard to adolescents, both the American Academy of Pediatrics (AAP) and Society for Adolescent Health and Medicine (SAHM) have released policy statements supporting minor consent for contraception.[3,4] As noted by SAHM, "The concepts of consent and confidentiality are inextricably intertwined. First, when a minor's own consent for health care is not legally sufficient, the process of obtaining consent from someone else compromises confidentiality. ... A legal basis for minors to consent to their own care also provides a strong foundation for protecting the confidentiality of the care."[4]

In spite of the widespread recognition of its importance, there is no United States (US) federal law or policy concerning adolescents' ability to consent for contraceptive services. In 1977, in *Carey v. Population Services International,* the Supreme Court expanded the right to obtain and use contraceptives to include minors. Overall, the guidance for minors' ability to consent for medical care, with or without specific provisions for contraception, defaults to state or local statutes. It is important that health care clinicians understand local laws and exemptions concerning minors' consent for contraception. Currently in the United States, 21 states and the District of Columbia explicitly allow all minors to consent to contraceptive services, and 25 states explicitly permit minors to consent to contraceptive services under specific circumstances.[5] In some states, there may be no explicit laws concerning minors' consent for contraception, or contraceptive services may fall under the statutes of general minors' consent for health care; however, funding for medical services may then determine minors' abilities to consent for contraception.

The Federal Title X Family Planning Program, established in 1970, requires adolescents' ability to consent for *confidential* contraceptive services, regardless of age.[6] In 2014, the Office of Population Health reaffirmed these provisions, including requirements to encourage family participation in the decision of minors to seek family planning services, and to provide counseling on how to resist attempts to coerce minors into engaging in sexual activities.[7] In addition, all Title X providers must comply with states' laws requiring notification or the reporting of child abuse, child molestation, sexual abuse, rape, and incest.[7] The federal Medicaid program requires family planning services be provided to beneficiaries, including "adolescents who can be deemed to be sexually active."[8] Medicaid also includes confidentiality protections.[8,9] Family planning services are available through comprehensive Medicaid, as are additional family planning–dedicated Medicaid programs (state family planning waiver programs) that include these requirements.[10] Comprehensive up-to-date summary of minors' consent laws are available on the Guttmacher Institute Web site.

MINOR CONSENT IN CASES OF GOVERNMENT CUSTODY

States may have separate requirements for minors in juvenile justice programs or under the custody of child protection services. The National Commission on Correctional Health Care recommends that incarcerated juveniles receive contraception and age-appropriate contraceptive information at an appropriate time before discharge, in accordance with local laws.[11] The 2015 guidance recommends women (including minor females) be provided with non-directive contraception counseling, access to emergency contraception (EC), and continuation of current contraceptive method while they are incarcerated.[12] In addition, the AAP recommends youth incarcerated for more than 1 week or in longer-term facilities receive comprehensive pediatric and adolescent preventive services.[13]

For youth involved with child protection services, the AAP recommends that "Safe, reliable birth control, ideally in the form of long-acting reversible contraception, should be made available."[14] Many localities have provisions that allow minors in state or county custody to consent for contraceptive services.[15] The National Campaign to Prevent Teen and Unintended Pregnancy and the National Council of Juvenile and Family Court Judges have developed a tool kit for system-involved youth entitled, "When You Decide: A Judge's Guide to Pregnancy Prevention Among Foster Youth With Bench Tools and Scripts."[16]

ADOLESCENT CONFIDENTIALITY

As noted in the SAHM statement, adolescents' right to consent and confidentiality in health care are intertwined. Providing confidentiality supports adolescents in their development of autonomy and plays a significant role in their willingness to access necessary health care or disclose important information with health care clinicians. The importance of confidentiality protections has been outlined by numerous international and national organizations. including the United Nations, SAHM, AAP, American Academy of Family Physicians (AAFP), and American College of Obstetricians and Gynecologists (ACOG).[17-21]

No federal law specifically guarantees the confidentiality of contraception or sexual health services for all minors. Specific federally funded family planning programs, such as Medicaid, Title X, and Medicaid waiver programs, provide individual protections for confidential access to contraception. Minor adolescents who receive contraception services through these funding programs receive confidentiality protections for information related to these services.[6,7] The 2002 federal guidance concerning the Health Insurance Portability and Accountability Act (HIPAA) also addressed the issue of minors' confidentiality. To summarize, the 2002 rule defers to any individual state protections of minors' confidentiality but states, "when a minor consents to a health care service and no other consent is required by law, if the minor voluntarily chooses to involve a parent or other adult, the minor nonetheless maintains the exclusive ability to exercise their rights under the rule. This is true even if a parent or other person also has consented to the health care service for which the minor lawfully consented."[22] In other words, if a minor has the right to consent to the services, the minor also has the right to confidentiality with regard to those services. Under the rule, a minor may involve a parent and still preserve the confidentiality of their protected health information.[22] The implication of this rule is that in states with specific laws allowing minor consent, adolescents may receive additional confidentiality protections. In states with no additional laws, the federal rules place the choice to provide or deny access (of information) to a parent under the discretion of a licensed health care professional, in the exercise of professional judgment.[23] Additionally, HIPAA protects confidentiality when a minor obtains care at the direction of a court or when a parent agrees that a health care clinicians and minor may have a confidential relationship.[17]

CONFIDENTIALITY CHALLENGES IN ELECTRONIC MEDICAL RECORDS AND INSURANCE BILLING

The expansion of electronic medical records and the increased coverage of young adults (up to age 26) through their parents' insurance plans have presented additional challenges to confidentiality. Although HIPAA provides security of protected health information from some disclosures, it also allows disclosure of information for the purpose of "treatment, payment, or healthcare operations" with consent.[22] Most health care clinicians probably are familiar with standard HIPAA privacy notices, seeking to obtain this consent from patients before they receive a service. Although a patient seeking a service may decline to sign the HIPAA consent allowing for disclosure to a payer, the practice or health care clinicians could then ask for the patient to be responsible for the entire cost of that service. Because health plans are not required to obtain consent of individuals before disclosure, it is possible that breach of confidentiality may result from an attempt to collect payment for a service. Under the law, individuals may request that their health plan send information by alternative means or to an alternative address; however, plans may require that individuals be able to pay in full for services rendered and justify how the disclosure of the information could endanger them.[24]

Many young people are covered as dependents on health insurance plans obtained by their parents through employers. According to the US Department of Labor, most of these private sector health plans are governed by another federal law, the Employee Retirement Income Security Act of 1974 (ERISA).[25] In order to ensure that policyholders are aware of and able to challenge coverage decisions, ERISA mandates notices of a denial of any portion of a claim along with reasons for the denial. With regard to adolescents covered by public insurance, federal Medicaid statute does not require sending explanation of benefits forms (EOBs); however, Medicaid Managed Care Plans must take steps to verify that billed services were provided and must send notices when services are denied.[24] The entity or individual (eg, health care clinicians, patient, head of household) who must be notified of denials is not specified, however, and procedures vary by state.[24]

Confidentiality breaches may occur when insurers send EOBs or denials of claims to policyholders after anyone covered under their policy obtains care. These insurance documents may identify the individual who received care, the health care clinicians, and the type of care obtained. In order to minimize the potential confidentiality breeches for minors and other dependents in insurance billing, 13 states have made provisions that serve to protect the confidentiality of individuals insured as dependents.[26] The specific provisions vary by state and include ability to request confidential communications, eliminating the requirements for EOBs to be sent, and mechanisms for EOBs to be sent to patients and not the policyholder. Even with these provisions in law, implementation is challenging, and the effect on adolescents is not always clear.[27] A summary of state provisions may be found at the Guttmacher Institute Web site.[26]

In 2016, AAP and SAHM released a joint policy statement on the importance of confidentiality protections in the insurance billing process. The statement indicates, "Policies and procedures should be established to ensure that health care billing and insurance claims processes such as explanation of benefit (EOB) notifications do not impede the confidential provision of health care services to adolescents and young adults.... Sending of EOBs or other similar notices should not be required when individuals insured as dependents obtain sensitive services." [28] In a separate statement, ACOG recommends, "Health care providers and institutions establishing an electronic health record (EHR) system should consider systems with adolescent-specific modules that can be customized to accommodate the confidentiality needs related to minor adolescents and comply with the requirements of state and federal laws. If the EHR system does not allow for procedures to maintain adolescent confidentiality, the health care provider or staff should inform the patient that parents will have access to the records, and the patient should be given the option for referral to a health care provider who is required to provide confidential care."[29] The AAP also has recommended confidentiality protections in its statement "Standards for Health Information Technology to Ensure Adolescent Privacy."[30]

EVIDENCE FOR THE EFFECTS OF CONSENT AND CONFIDENTIALITY LAWS ON CONTRACEPTIVE ACCESS AND ADOLESCENT HEALTH

Despite the widely recognized importance of adolescent confidentiality, research shows that minor adolescents and young adults continue to encounter substantial barriers to confidential contraceptive services. In 2017, Fuentes et al[31] found that confidentiality concerns among both sexually experienced adolescent and young adult women were associated with a significantly reduced likelihood of having received a contraceptive service. Among sexually experienced girls aged 15 to 17 years, 22% of those with confidentiality concerns received any contraceptive services compared to 67% of those who did not report concerns. Among sexually experienced 18- to 25-year-old women, 47% of those reporting confidentiality concerns received any contraceptive service in the past year compared to 75% of those who reported none.[31] Overall, adolescents and young adults entitled to services through Medicaid and Title X programs accessed more resources as they had significantly less concerns about confidentiality. The study by Fuentes et al[31] also found 1 in 10 young adults aged 18 to 25 years on their parents' health insurance and nearly 1 in 5 of all adolescents aged 15 to 17 years reported that they would not seek sexual and reproductive health care services because of concerns that their parents might find out.

There is ample evidence on the health effects of the ability to self-consent/assent on adolescents' health and well-being. In states that have greater access to contraception, the teen birthrate is significant lower than in states with less access.[32] For example, Massachusetts has the lowest teen birthrate (8.5 per 1000),[33] allows all minor adolescents to consent for all family planning services (with the exception of sterilization or abortion),[34] has the most comprehensive confidentiality protections for adolescent minors,[34] and has the lowest uninsured rate in the United States.[35] Texas has limited minors' consent for contraception (federal programs and minors in custody only),[36] has the highest uninsured rate (15%),[36] has no state confidentiality protections, and has a teen birthrate of 31.0 per 1000 (nearly 400% the Massachusetts rate).[37] Providers may access training and resources to provide confidential reproductive health care through the Confidential and Covered Project.[27]

CONTRACEPTION AFFORDABILITY AND EQUITY

Access to affordable contraception is crucial for adolescents' health and well-being, especially to prevent unintended pregnancies and teen births. In the United States, publicly supported family planning efforts save $7.09 for every $1 spent, with most of the cost recovery deriving from preventing unplanned births.[38] Implementation of the Affordable Care Act (ACA) greatly expanded financial access to contraception because it requires health insurance coverage for the full range of US Food and Drug Administration (FDA)-approved contraceptive methods (18 specific methods) used by women without out-of-pocket costs.[39] States have their own requirements that provide additional guarantees in the event of exceptions to the federal mandate or future erosions of the ACA requirements. The Guttmacher Institute maintains a current summary of these laws.[40] The ACA mandate has significantly benefited women, especially adolescents and low-wage earners. The National Women's Law Center estimates that 62.4 million women have insurance coverage of birth control without out-of-pocket costs as of 2017.[41] A 2015 Health Affairs study found the average contraceptive pill user saved $255 per year, and the average intrauterine device user saved $250 per year after the ACA mandate took effect.[42] Canestaro et al[43] found that the long-term gains of affordable contraception were important in terms of preventing more costly outcomes. They found providing no contraception coverage resulted in 33 more unintended pregnancies per 1000 women and significantly increased the number of unintended births and terminations.[43] Total costs were higher among uninsured women because of the higher costs of pregnancy outcomes.[43]

In spite of well-researched evidence of large societal and individual savings, improved health outcomes, and significant public support, contraception coverage remains threatened.[44,45] Several high-profile lawsuits and administrative policies have eroded coverage for employees if employers have religious or moral objections to the contraceptive services, even if the employers' insurance plans are not directly paying for the services.[46] Many medical and health organizations, including AAP and SAHM, oppose these exceptions to contraceptive coverage.[47,48] Providers may assist patients with contraceptive coverage through the National Women's Law Center's Cover Her campaign.[49] This campaign includes a hotline for patients and providers to contact for assistance with no out-of-pocket payments for contraception access and a college campus toolkit. The National Health Law Program also provides resources for state-level advocacy to provide contraception access protection.[50]

NON-PRESCRIPTION ACCESS TO HORMONAL AND EMERGENCY CONTRACEPTION

An additional strategy to increase the availability of contraception is non-prescription access. An important example of this approach is over-the-counter (OTC) levonorgestrel EC. After a delay of 10 years from the initial recommendation of the FDA advisory panel, OTC EC was released for distribution without age restriction in 2013[51,52]; however, OTC status does not eliminate access barriers. Research by the Society for Emergency Contraception continues to document age restrictions implemented by retailers, inconsistent in-store availability, and high costs; however, despite persistent barriers since approval, the rate of EC use, including among adolescents, has increased significantly.[53]

Currently no daily oral contraceptive pill is approved for OTC use in the United States. Studies are currently underway as part of an application to the FDA to switch a progestin-only daily contraceptive pill from prescription to OTC status. Such FDA approval without an age restriction is questionable given the history of OTC EC. Many provider and women's health organizations have signed on to the Oral Contraceptives Over-the-Counter Working Group Statement of Purpose in support of efforts to bring oral contraception OTC without age restriction,[54] and some policymakers have endorsed legislation that would allow OTC access to those 18 years and older.[55]

An intermediate step between clinic/prescription and OTC access is pharmacy provision. In this model, which has been implemented in some states including Oregon and California, pharmacists are authorized to provide hormonal contraceptives directly to consumers, without requiring visits to the health care provider first. The range of options available can vary to include oral formulations only or may include other delivery mechanisms such as the patch or injectables. The Association of State and Territorial Health Officials tracks state policies regarding pharmacist provision of contraception on their Web site (www.astho.org/state-legislative-tracking/). As with other innovations to expand contraceptive access, pharmacy provision policies have benefits and limitations. A potential benefit for access is the ubiquitous nature of pharmacies in communities along with potentially more extensive hours of operation (ie, nights and weekends) compared with clinics. On the other hand, previous experience with pharmacy access to EC models did show that some pharmacists were unwilling to provide EC to minors because of personal beliefs and despite regulations.[56] Cost of services and ability to confidentially bill insurance through the pharmacy are other potential barriers limiting the willingness of adolescents to access contraception in pharmacy settings.

CONSCIENTIOUS OBJECTIONS AND THE RESPONSIBILITIES OF THE CLINICIAN

Another barrier adolescents may face in accessing contraception is the conscientious objections of their health care providers, which may occur when physicians have moral objections to certain medical treatments. Conscientious objections may include omissions of complete discussion of methods, denial of confidentiality, coercion toward certain methods, and refusal to write prescriptions. These barriers leave adolescents without the full range of contraceptive services, therefore denying their rights to voluntary, comprehensive, informed health care decisions. Even though most Americans support contraception services, policymakers have used moral arguments to restrict access to contraception. The Obama administration initially blocked OTC sale of levonorgestrel-based EC without age restrictions despite full FDA approval for OTC use without restrictions.[57] Most recently, the Trump administration issued a rule that expanded exemptions to protect religious and moral convictions for certain entities and individuals whose health plans are subject to a mandate of contraceptive coverage.[58] Another rule allows a broad range of health care practitioners to opt out of providing care based on the grounds of conscientious objection without any obligation to refer patients to a source that may provide the necessary or desired services.[59]

The AAP policy statement "Physician Refusal to Provide Information or Treatment on the Basis of Claims of Conscience" acknowledges the importance of balancing respect for the health care clinicians' right to their moral conscience, the moral obligation to inform their patients of relevant alternatives as part of the informed consent process, and the duty to refer patients who desire these treatments in a timely manner when failing to do so would harm the patients.[60] Furthermore, APHA supports the right of all individuals to evidence-based, comprehensive contraceptive counseling and education free from personal bias, including information on the risks, benefits, effectiveness, proper usage, alternatives, and adverse effects, accompanied by a comprehensible, culturally/linguistically appropriate informed consent process. The APHA also advocates for measures that ensure implementation of referral systems for contraceptive services in cases of conscientious objection.[2] Providers can find resources for advocacy at the Reproductive Health Access Project and Physicians for Reproductive Health.[61,62]

SUMMARY

Laws and policies regarding consent, confidentiality, cost of contraception, and conscientious objections have significant effects on adolescents' abilities to access reproductive health services. The landscape of policies is dynamic, and it is important for providers to stay well informed of current laws and proposed changes. Public health organizations, professional societies, and interest groups provide guidance and resources that facilitate providers advocating for their patients to access confidential and affordable contraceptive care.

QUESTIONS

1. A 17-year-old female patient presents to the clinic by herself and requests contraception. Her ability to consent to receive contraception as a minor is:
   A. Protected by the federal Title X statute.
   B. Dependent on the law in her state.
   C. Guaranteed under the federal Health Insurance Portability and Protection Act (HIPAA) statute.
   D. Protected by United Nations policy.

2. An 18-year-old female college student presents to a Title X clinic requesting contraceptive care. She is covered as a dependent on her parent's private insurance plan. She thinks the plan covers contraception but doesn't want her parents to know about it and asks whether it is possible for her information to remain confidential. The best response to her question is:
   A. The American Academy of Pediatrics and the Society for Adolescent Health and Medicine have stated that confidentiality in the insurance billing and claims process is vital and that she can use her insurance without disclosing her information to her parents.
   B. The Title X statute is designed to ensure affordable access to family planning services, including contraception, and provides for the ability to bill her insurance plan confidentially.
   C. If her plan covers contraception the service should be paid for, but if her insurance is billed, the plan's notices regarding use of benefits could be sent to the policyholder.
   D. The HIPAA statute guarantees her right to privacy regarding her health care when using her insurance plan.
3. Non-prescription access to hormonal contraception is one approach to increasing access for individuals, including adolescents. Non-prescription access includes pharmacists dispensing hormonal contraception to patients without clinical visits first and over-the-counter (OTC) contraception products. Currently in the United States:
   A. Levonorgestrel and ulipristal emergency contraceptive pills are available OTC throughout the United States by Food and Drug Administration (FDA) approval.
   B. State laws permitting pharmacy access to hormonal contraception have been implemented in several states, including Oregon and California.
   C. The FDA regulations permit OTC sales of levonorgestrel emergency contraception for adults 18 years and older but not to minors.

(See page 204 for answers.)

References

1. United Nations Population Fund, Center for Reproductive Rights. Briefing paper: the rights to contraceptive information and services for women and adolescents. Center for Reproductive Rights. https://www.unfpa.org/sites/default/files/resource-pdf/Contraception.pdf. Accessed January 4, 2019
2. American Public Health Association. Universal access to contraception. https://www.apha.org/policies-and-advocacy/public-health-policy-statements/policy-database/2015/12/17/09/14/universal-access-to-contraception. Updated November 3, 2015. Accessed June 15, 2018
3. Ott MA, Sucato GS; American Academy of Pediatrics Committee on Adolescence. Contraception for adolescents. *Pediatrics*. 2014;134(4):e1257-e1281
4. Ford C, English A, Sigman G. Confidential health care for adolescents: position paper for the Society for Adolescent Medicine. *J Adolesc Health*. 2004;35(2):160-167
5. Guttmacher Institute. Minors' access to contraception. https://www.guttmacher.org/state-policy/explore/minors-access-contraceptive-services. Updated 2018. Accessed June 20, 2018
6. Department of Health and Human Services Office of Population Affairs. Program requirements for Title X funded family planning projects. https://www.hhs.gov/opa/sites/default/files/Title-X-2014-Program-Requirements.pdf. Updated April 2014. Accessed June 13, 2018

7. Department of Health and Human Services Office of Population Affairs. OPA program policy notice 2014-01—Confidential services to adolescents. https://www.hhs.gov/opa/sites/default/files/ppn2014-01-001.pdf. Published June 5, 2014. Accessed June 13, 2018
8. Summers R. CMS advancements in Medicaid family planning. https://www.nationalfamilyplanning.org/file/NFPRHA-Medicaid-Family-Planning-Interested-Parties-Memo---August-2016.pdf. Updated 2016. Accessed June 14, 2018
9. English A. Adolescent confidentiality protections in Title X. https://www.nationalfamilyplanning.org/document.doc?id=1559. Updated 2015. Accessed June 14, 2018
10. Kaiser Family Foundation. Medicaid and family planning: background and implications of the ACA. https://www.kff.org/report-section/medicaid-and-family-planning-medicaid-family-planning-policy/. Updated 2016. Accessed June 15, 2018
11. National Conference of State Legislatures. Medicaid for juvenile justice involved children. 2015. http://www.ncsl.org/documents/cj/jjguidebook-medicaid.pdf. Accessed November 21, 2018
12. National Commission on Correctional Health Care. Women's health care in correctional settings. https://www.ncchc.org/womens-health-care. Updated 2014. Accessed June 15, 2018
13. American Academy of Pediatrics Committee on Adolescence. Health care for youth in the juvenile justice system. *Pediatrics*. 2011;128(6):1219-1235
14. American Academy of Pediatrics Council on Foster Care, Adoption, and Kinship Care, Committee on Adolescence, Council on Early Childhood. Health care issues for children and adolescents in foster care and kinship care. *Pediatrics*. 2015;136(4):1131-e1140
15. Reilly C. For foster teens, accessing birth control is an uphill battle. Rewire News. December 20, 2017. https://rewire.news/article/2017/12/20/foster-teens-accessing-birth-control-uphill-battle/. Accessed June 16, 2018
16. Escher P, Whitney Barnes E. When you decide: a judge's guide to pregnancy prevention among foster youth with bench tools and scripts. The National Campaign to Prevent Teen and Unplanned Pregnancy. September 2015. https://powertodecide.org/what-we-do/information/resource-library/when-you-decide. Accessed January 4, 2019
17. Standards for privacy of individually identifiable health information. Office of the Assistant Secretary for Planning and Evaluation, DHHS. Final rule. *Fed Regist*. 2000;65(250):82462-82829
18. Department of Health and Human Services. Does the HIPAA privacy rule allow parents the right to see their children's medical records? https://www.hhs.gov/hipaa/for-professionals/faq/227/can-i-access-medical-record-if-i-have-power-of-attorney/index.html. Published December 19, 2002. Accessed June 21, 2018
19. American Academy of Pediatrics. Confidentiality laws tip sheet. https://www.aap.org/en-us/advocacy-and-policy/aap-health-initiatives/healthy-foster-care-america/Documents/Confidentiality_Laws.pdf. Accessed January 4, 2019
20. de Crombrugghe B. Report of the human rights council on its thirty-second session. United Nations. 2016. https://www.ohchr.org/EN/HRBodies/HRC/RegularSessions/Session32/Documents/A.HRC.32.2_AUV.doc. Accessed November 21, 2018
21. Marcell AV, Burstein GR; American Academy of Pediatrics Committee on Adolescence. Sexual and reproductive health care services in the pediatric setting. *Pediatrics*. 2017;140(5):e20172858
22. American Academy of Family Physicians. Adolescent health care, confidentiality. https://www.aafp.org/about/policies/all/adolescent-confidentiality.html. Updated 1988. Accessed June 23, 2018
23. American College of Obstetricians and Gynecologists. Committee on Adolescent Health Care. Committee Opinion No. 710: Counseling adolescents about contraception. *Obstet Gynecol*. 2017;130(2):e74-e80
24. National Health Law Program. Webinar confidentiality: implications for access to sexual and reproductive health care, March 11, 2016. https://healthlaw.org/resource/webinar-confidentiality-protections-implications-on-access-to-sexual-and-reproductive-health-care/. Accessed November 21, 2018
25. US Department of Labor. Health plans and benefits. https://www.dol.gov/general/topic/health-plans. Accessed September 28, 2018
26. Guttmacher Institute. Protecting confidentiality for individuals insured as dependents. https://www.guttmacher.org/state-policy/explore/protecting-confidentiality-individuals-insured-dependents. Updated 2018. Accessed June 23, 2019

27. National Family Planning and Reproductive Health Association. Confidential and covered. https://www.nationalfamilyplanning.org/confidentialandcovered. Accessed January 4, 2019
28. Society for Adolescent Health and Medicine, American Academy of Pediatrics. Confidentiality protections for adolescents and young adults in the health care billing and insurance claims process. *J Adolesc Health.* 2016;58(3):374-377
29. ACOG Committee Opinion No. 599: Committee on adolescent health care: adolescent confidentiality and electronic health records. *Obstet Gynecol.* 2014;123(5):1148-1150
30. American Academy of Pediatrics Committee on Adolescence, Council on Clinical and Information Technology; Blythe MJ, Del Beccaro MA. Standards for health information technology to ensure adolescent privacy. *Pediatrics.* 2012;130(5):987-990
31. Fuentes L, Ingerick M, Jones R, Lindberg L. Adolescents' and young adults' reports of barriers to confidential health care and receipt of contraceptive services. *J Adolesc Health.* 2018;62(1):36-43
32. Lindberg L, Santelli J, Desai S. Understanding the decline in adolescent fertility in the United States, 2007-2012. *J Adolesc Health.* 2016;59(5):577-583
33. Centers for Disease Control and Prevention. Stats of the state of Massachusetts. https://www.cdc.gov/nchs/pressroom/sosmap/teen-births/teenbirths.htm. Updated 2018. Accessed June 23, 2018
34. Boston College Law School Juvenile Rights Advocacy Project. Consent to medical treatment by minors in Massachusetts: a guide for practitioners. Juvenile Rights Advocacy Project. 2006. https://www.bc.edu/content/dam/files/schools/law_sites/jrap/pdf/jrap_medical_consent.pdf. Accessed June 23, 2018
35. Kaiser Family Foundation. Health insurance coverage of the total population. https://www.kff.org/other/state-indicator/total-population/?currentTimeframe=0&sortModel=%7B%22colId%22:%22Uninsured%22,%22sort%22:%22desc%22%7D. Accessed June 24, 2018
36. Guttmacher Institute. An overview of minors' consent laws. https://www.guttmacher.org/state-policy/explore/overview-minors-consent-law. Updated 2018. Accessed June 23, 2018
37. The National Campaign to Prevent Teen and Unintended Pregnancy. Teen birth rate among girls age 15-19. https://powertodecide.org/what-we-do/information/national-state-data/teen-birth-rate. Accessed June 23, 2018
38. Frost JJ, Sonfield A, Zolna MR, Finer LB. Return on investment: a fuller assessment of the benefits and cost savings of the US publicly funded family planning program. *Milbank Q.* 2014;92(4):696-749
39. US Food and Drug Administration. Birth control chart. https://www.fda.gov/forconsumers/byaudience/forwomen/freepublications/ucm522453.htm. Updated February 16, 2018. Accessed June 23, 2018
40. Guttmacher Institute. Insurance coverage of contraceptives. https://www.guttmacher.org/state-policy/explore/insurance-coverage-contraceptives. Updated 2018. Accessed June 23, 2018
41. National Women's Law Center. New data estimate 62.4 million women have coverage of birth control without out-of-pocket costs. https://nwlc.org/resources/new-data-estimate-62-4-million-women-have-coverage-of-birth-control-without-out-of-pocket-costs/. Updated 2017. Accessed June 24, 2018
42. Becker NV, Polsky D. Women saw large decrease in out-of-pocket spending for contraceptives after ACA mandate removed cost sharing. *Health Aff (Millwood).* 2015;34(7):1204-1211
43. Canestaro W, Vodicka E, Downing D, Trussell J. Implications of employer coverage of contraception: cost-effectiveness analysis of contraception coverage under an employer mandate. *Contraception.* 2017;95(1):77-89
44. PerryUndem. Contraceptives and policy through a gender lens. March 22, 2017. https://www.scribd.com/document/342699692/PerryUndem-Gender-and-Birth-Control-Access-Report. Accessed November 21, 2018
45. Sobel L, Salganicoff A, Rosenzweig C. The future of contraceptive coverage. https://www.kff.org/womens-health-policy/issue-brief/the-future-of-contraceptive-coverage/. Henry J. Kaiser Family Foundation Web site. Published January 9, 2017. Accessed June 24, 2018
46. Goldstein A, Eilperin J, Wan W. Trump administration narrows Affordable Care Act's contraception mandate. *Washington Post.* October 6, 2017. https://www.washingtonpost.com/national/health-science/trump-administration-could-narrow-affordable-care-acts-contraception-

mandate/2017/10/05/16139400-a9f0-11e7-92d1-58c702d2d975_story.html?noredirect=on&utm_term=.6081cab59967. Accessed June 24, 2018
47. American Academy of Pediatrics. New Trump administration rules limiting contraception access jeopardize health of adolescents, women and families. https://www.aap.org/en-us/about-the-aap/aap-press-room/Pages/AAPSAHMContraceptiveRule.aspx. Updated October 6, 2017. Accessed June 24, 2018
48. Society for Adolescent Health and Medicine. SAHM statement regarding contraceptive access policies. https://www.adolescenthealth.org/SAHM_Main/media/Advocacy/2017%20sign%20on/SAHM-Statement-Regarding-Contraceptive-Access-Policies.pdf. Updated 2017. Accessed June 24, 2018
49. National Women's Law Center. CoverHer. https://nwlc.org/coverher/. Accessed June 24, 2018
50. National Health Law Program. Fact sheet: State contraceptive equity laws. https://healthlaw.org/resource/fact-sheet-state-contraceptive-equity-laws/. Updated January 29, 2018. Accessed November 26, 2018
51. History of Plan B OTC. The Emergency Contraception Website. http://ec.princeton.edu/pills/planbhistory.html. Accessed November 26, 2018
52. Sifferlin A. Timeline: the battle for plan B. Time Magazine Web site. http://healthland.time.com/2013/06/11/timeline-the-battle-for-plan-b/. Updated June 11, 2013. Accessed June 28, 2018
53. Martinez GM, Abma JC. Sexual activity, contraceptive use, and childbearing of teenagers aged 15-19 in the United States. *NCHS Data Brief.* 2015;209:1-8
54. Oral Contraceptives Over-the-Counter Working Group. Statement of purpose. http://ocsotc.org/statement-of-purpose/. Accessed November 26, 2018
55. Ayotte, Gardner introduce bill aimed at increasing availability of safe and effective over-the-counter contraceptives. United States Senator Cory Gardner Web site. https://www.gardner.senate.gov/newsroom/press-releases/ayotte-gardner-introduce-bill-aimed-at-increasing-availability-of-safe-and-effective-over-the-counter-contraceptives. Published May 21, 2015. Accessed June 30, 2018
56. Conard LA, Fortenberry JD, Blythe MJ, Orr DP. Pharmacists' attitudes toward and practices with adolescents. *Arch Pediatr Adolesc Med.* 2003;157(4):361-365
57. Rowan A. Obama administration yields to the courts and the evidence, allows emergency contraception to be sold without restrictions. https://www.guttmacher.org/gpr/2013/06/obama-administration-yields-courts-and-evidence-allows-emergency-contraception-be-sold. Published June 25, 2013. Accessed June 24, 2018
58. Internal Revenue Service, Department of the Treasury, Employee Benefits Security Administration, Department of Labor, Centers for Medicare & Medicaid Services, Department of Health and Human Services. Moral exemptions and accommodations for coverage of certain preventive services under the Affordable Care Act. *Fed Regist.* 2017;82(197):47838-47862
59. Department of Health and Human Services. Protecting statutory conscience rights in health care; delegations of authority. *Federal Register.* https://www.federalregister.gov/documents/2018/01/26/2018-01226/protecting-statutory-conscience-rights-in-health-care-delegations-of-authority. Accessed June 26, 2018
60. Committee on Bioethics. Policy statement—physician refusal to provide information or treatment on the basis of claims of conscience. *Pediatrics.* 2009;124(6):1689-1693
61. Reproductive Health Access Project. Clinician advocacy. https://www.reproductiveaccess.org/get-involved/mobilize/clinician-advocacy/. Accessed November 26, 2018
62. Physicians for Reproductive Health. https://prh.org/. Accessed October 3, 2018

Adolesc Med 030 (2019) 187–195

New Contraceptive Developments on the Horizon

Orquidia Torres, MD, MS[a*]; Elizabeth Alderman, MD[b]

[a]*Assistant Professor of Pediatrics, Department of Pediatrics, Division of Adolescent Medicine, Children's Hospital at Montefiore, Bronx, New York;* [b]*Professor of Pediatrics, Department of Pediatrics, Division of Adolescent Medicine, Children's Hospital at Montefiore, Bronx, New York*

LEARNING OBJECTIVES

After reviewing this article, the reader should be able to:

1. Identify new contraceptive options being researched for men and women
2. Compare the mechanism of action between current and new contraceptives
3. Critique the applicability of new contraceptives in adolescents

INTRODUCTION

Unintended adolescent pregnancy rates have declined in the United States (US).[1] Moreover, the rate of abortion has also decreased in this time frame.[1] Despite this decrease, the United States has one of the highest rates of adolescent pregnancy among the developed countries.[1] The decline in pregnancy can be attributed to the availability and acceptance of contraception, particularly of less user-dependent forms of contraception such as the implant and the intrauterine device (IUD).[2] Although contraceptive rates among adolescents in the United States have increased over time, sexual activity rates have remained the same.[2]

Long-acting reversible contraception (LARC), which are IUDs and implants, are the most effective forms of contraception and are recommended as first-line contraception by the American College of Obstetricians and Gynecologists and the American Academy of Pediatrics.[3,4] Use of LARC in the US increased to 8% from 2011 to 2015 for females aged 15 to 44 years, but adolescents continue to use other forms of contraception at higher rates.[5] Worldwide, LARC use is about

*Corresponding author
E-mail address: ortorres@montefiore.org

 ISSN 1934-4287

14%, with Asia having the highest rates of IUD use.[6,7] About 10% of women worldwide have an unmet need for contraception.[6] Cultural norms, cost, and access have contributed to this unmet need. New contraceptive options aim to improve cost and access in developing countries.

Although several contraceptive options are available today, it took decades for different contraceptives to be developed and approved in the United States in the setting of controversial political restrictions. These restrictions came into effect after the first oral contraceptive pills were approved by the US Food and Drug Administration (FDA) in 1960.[8] Women, both married and unmarried, were denied access because of societal beliefs at the time. Side effects have also affected the interest in and continuation of use of certain contraceptives.

In the 1990s, Norplant (1990), Depo-Provera (1992), the female condom (1993), and Plan B One-Step (1999) were approved by the FDA.[8] In the 2000s, Ortho Evra (2001), NuvaRing (2001), improved female condoms (2009), and ulipristal acetate (2010) were introduced.[8] By 2002, Norplant was discontinued in the United States, and single-rod etonogestrel implants were later approved. Nexplanon (2011) replaced Implanon (2006).[8] After the removal of the Dalkon Shield from the market in the 1970s, it took about 3 decades for other IUDs to be approved: ParaGard in 1998 and Mirena in 2000.[9] Twelve years after the release of Mirena, another hormonal IUD, Skyla, was introduced.[8] The last contraceptive approved in the United States was the hormonal IUD Kyleena in 2016.[9]

The United States has come a long way in the acceptance of birth control, but further research is needed to improve certain aspects of contraception. Many of the new contraceptives are in development in other countries besides the US. Current advances, described in this article, aim to change the side effect profiles and delivery of current contraceptives. Moreover, the need to develop more reliable and less user-dependent contraception that can be used by adolescent boys would provide more choices and possibly empower adolescent boys to take a role in prevention of unintended pregnancy.

NEW CONTRACEPTIVE DEVELOPMENTS FOR FEMALES

Variant of Existing Forms of Contraception

A subcutaneous form of medroxyprogesterone acetate, DMPA-SC, is administered every 3 months. It is manufactured as depo-subQ provera 104 in the US and as Sayana Press in other countries.[10] Sayana Press (Figure 1) is approved and available in several European and African countries. Self-injection of DMPA-SC was approved in 2015 in the United Kingdom by the Medicares and Health Care Products Regulatory Agency and recommended by the World Health Organization.[11] A funding collaboration has helped to price DMPA-SC at $1 per dose.[11] DMPA-SC is available via Uniject, an injection system that can be used for self-

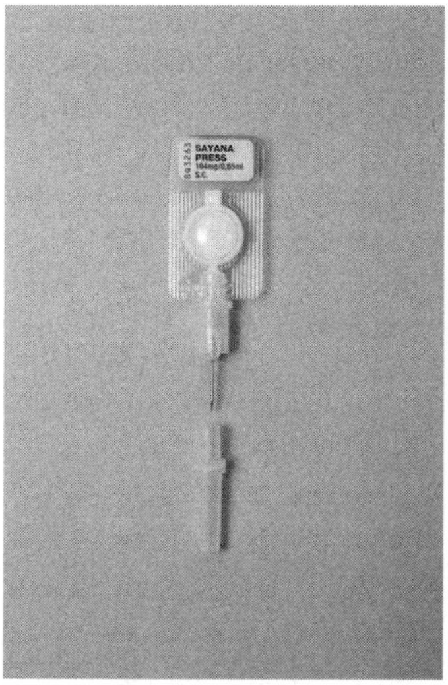

Fig 1. The injectable contraceptive subcutaneous medroxyprogesterone acetate (DMPA-SC or brand name Sayana Press) in the BD Uniject injection system.
© 2013 PATH/Patrick McKern, Courtesy of Photoshare.

administration.[11] Uniject has a single dose of the medication in a plastic blister.[10] The subcutaneous formulation allows for it to be absorbed slowly, so a lower dose is required.[10] DMPA-SC is as safe and effective as injectable medroxyprogesterone acetate, with similar side effects of weight gain, menstrual irregularities, and headaches.[10] The advantages of DMPA-SC are use of shorter needles and fewer risks compared to intramuscular injections.[10] Therefore, health care team members require a lower level of training to administer the medication. Research involving self-injection of DMPA-SC in Uganda and Senegal has shown promising results, with 90% of the participants proficient with the injection after training.[12] Self-injection with DMPA-SC in adolescents in Uganda revealed that the majority felt it was a timesaving, cost-effective, and discreet contraceptive.[13]

The FDA approved female condoms in the United States in the early 1990s.[8] The Female Health Company transitioned from polyurethane female condoms to non-polyurethane FC2 female condoms to lower costs.[14] With this transition, sales of FC2 condoms increased.[14] Since the early 2000s, other female condoms have been developed to improve their functionality and cost.[14] Several versions of the female condom are on the market now in different countries.[14]

Contraception Development in Progress

In 2012, the Bill and Melinda Gates Foundation provided funding for a company in Massachusetts, now named Keratin Biosciences, Inc. (formerly Microchips

Biotech), to develop a microchip hormonal implant.[15] The microchip contains levonorgestrel, enough to last 16 years, and measures 20 × 20 × 7 mm.[16] Levonorgestrel is embedded in a hermetic titanium and platinum seal on the reservoirs of the device.[15,16] A small amount of the hormone is released daily when electric current passes through the seal.[16] The device can be remotely controlled by the patient or physician through wireless remote.[15] Essentially, women would be able to control the device when they are ready to conceive. Because it functions wirelessly, the device is encrypted.[15] The microchip hormonal implant is currently undergoing testing for safety and efficacy in the United States. The technology has already demonstrated success with delivering human parathyroid hormone in patients with osteoporosis.[17]

Currently, various refinements have been made to IUDs. VeraCept is a copper IUD currently being tested in phase 3 clinical trials in the US.[18] Compared to the copper IUD currently available in the US, VeraCept has a lower copper dosage, is composed of a flexible memory frame (nitinol), and has a smaller preloaded inserter with pretrimmed strings.[18] The memory frame is designed to change shape in relation to the uterus to reduce expulsion and cause less discomfort.[19] Research comparing VeraCept to the copper IUD in the US demonstrated less pain on insertion, lower expulsion rate, higher continuation rates (less removals because of bleeding and pain), and similar contraception effectiveness.[19]

LevoCept is a levonorgestrel-containing IUD that also has the memory frame and smaller preloaded inserter with precut strings.[20] LevoCept is in phase 2 of clinical trials.[20]

Another intrauterine contraceptive, the intrauterine ball (IUB), has a similar concept to VeraCept. It has slightly less copper, is composed of copper pearls, and is designed using the memory frame that takes a spherical form as opposed to the T configuration (Figure 2).[21] The IUB is effective in preventing pregnancy for 5 years.[21] IUB clinical trials in Romania, Bulgaria, and Hungary were done.

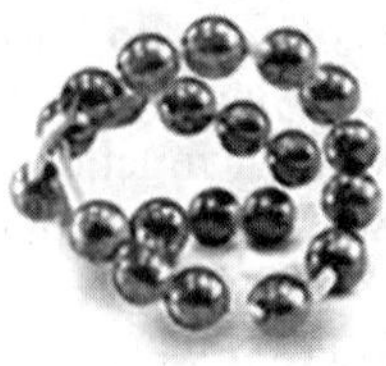

Fig 2. Intrauterine ball. Courtesy of OCON Medical.

Although the expectation for the IUB is lower rates of expulsion and perforation, research thus far shows high expulsion and discontinuation rates after 1 year.[22]

In China, other types of copper IUDs containing indomethacin have been developed. Studies have shown that patients have less bleeding and higher continuation rates with this type of IUD.[23] However, it has been demonstrated that patients have needed cervical dilation during insertion.[23]

In August 2018, the FDA approved a year-long intravaginal ring containing segesterone acetate and ethinyl estradiol.[24] This new form of contraception is placed in the vagina for 3 weeks and removed for 1 week for withdrawal bleeding.[24] The ring can be stored in a compact case and reused for the next cycle.[24] Bayer is also working on a year-long progestin-only vaginal ring containing levonorgestrel.[25] Another vaginal ring in the testing phases contains dapivirine and would provide both contraception and protection against human immunodeficiency virus. A phase 3 randomized controlled trial assessing the use the dapivirine vaginal ring in Malawi, South Africa, Uganda, and Zimbabwe demonstrated a decreased risk of human immunodeficiency virus-1 infection, particularly among those with increased adherence.[26]

All progestin-only pills in the US contain norethindrone. A French company, Leon Pharma, is testing a progestin-only pill containing drospirenone, the same progestin in Yaz and Yasmin.[25] A new contraceptive patch, Twirla, is also in development in the United States.[25] Phase 3 trials were completed, but Twirla has not been approved by the FDA yet.[25] Currently, Xulane is the only patch available. Twirla contains levonorgestrel as the progestin component, releases a smaller amount of estrogen per day, and uses a different adhesive that prevents the breakdown of adhesive at the edges of the patch.[25]

NEW CONTRACEPTIVE DEVELOPMENTS FOR MALES

Although condoms and sterilization have been the only forms of male contraception, new developments are underway, leading to the possibility that contraceptive decision-making and use would not be solely by the female. In the past, there has not been much development in male contraception because of minimal funding and the complexities of the male reproductive system.[27] Although male contraception is currently limited, research has shown that males would be interested in male hormonal contraception.[27]

Male Hormonal Contraception Development in Progress

The World Health Organization previously tested the use of testosterone enanthate weekly intramuscular injections as contraception in two international studies.[28] These studies revealed that testosterone can be used to achieve azoospermia and oligospermia.[28] Testosterone undecanoate, a testosterone injection used for replacement in hypogonadism, is being tested in China as a form of contraception.[27] The phase 3 trial in China showed 95% efficacy for pregnancy prevention with testosterone undecanoate, but it was not approved by the regulatory authorities.[27]

Transdermal testosterone and nestorone gel applied to male external genitalia has been studied in a multicenter randomized trial in the United States. The study demonstrated that the combination of testosterone and nestorone achieved azoospermia in 88.5% of participants.[27] Ongoing research is taking place to evaluate for potential side effects.

Male Non-Hormonal Contraception Development in Progress

Gendarussa, an herb that grows in Indonesia, has been researched as a male contraceptive agent. Gendarussa is proposed to affect sperm penetration of an ovum.[29] Only 1 pregnancy occurred during clinical phase trials in Indonesia.[29]

The "clean sheets" pill was developed by researchers in London.[29] It is hormone-free and inhibits the release of semen without affecting an orgasm.[29] It is based on phenoxybenzamine, which has the adverse effect of inhibiting ejaculation.[29] The pill can be taken up to 3 hours before intercourse and wears off within 16 to 24 hours.[29] It works by relaxing the muscles of the epididymis and vas deferens.[29] It also prevents secretion of fluid from accessory glands.[29] The pill could potentially reduce the transmission of sexually transmitted infections since no seminal fluid is released when using this contraceptive.[29] Nonetheless, this potential contraceptive still requires further testing in animals and humans.[29]

Gamendazole, a non-hormonal contraceptive pill, prohibits sperm from reaching maturity and allows reabsorption into the testes.[30] Animal testing demonstrated 100% infertility after 1 dose in rats, but only 57% reversible.[28] Further research is needed before this option is available for men.

Alternatives to Vasectomy in Progress

Longer-lasting contraception for men is being tested and developed. Vas-occlusion induces infertility essentially by blocking sperm transport. Various attempts with this method have been unsuccessful since the 1960s. Reversible inhibition of sperm under guidance (RISUG) is a form of vas-occlusion that requires injection of the polymer gel styrene maleic anhydride (SMA) into the vas deferens to form a blockage.[27,28] The gel can be expelled using solvent to flush it out and by electrical stimulation to cause contractions.[27] Clinical trials of RISUG in India have demonstrating pregnancy prevention for several years.[27] However, there are concerns for safety with this method. The polymer has pH-lowering effects that can damage sperm.[28] Trial data have also demonstrated sperm abnormalities, including bent and coiled tails and amorphous heads.[28] Studies of RISUG in Langur monkeys have shown vacuolization in Sertoli cells and shrunken seminiferous tubules.[28]

Vasalgel is being developed in the United States. Vasalgel is composed of the polymer styrene maleic acid dissolved in an organic solvent.[29] Unlike RISUG, Vasalgel is reported to have no sperm-altering effects.[28] Animal testing with monkeys have shown pregnancy prevention for up to 2 years with this method.[28]

Percutaneous injections of occlusive material into the vas deferens have also been researched because Vasalgel and RISUG require a surgical procedure. Percutaneous injection of polyurethane elastomer has been studied in China, and medical-grade silicone rubber has been studied in Indonesia and the Netherlands.[28] Males in these studies did achieve azoospermia, but issues remain with regard to the applicators and the timing required for the material to form inside the vas lumen.[28]

CONCLUSION

Numerous new contraceptive agents are in development. Contraceptive options such as DMPA-SC show promise for pregnancy prevention worldwide given its low cost and ease of use. New developments with IUDs can possibly help reduce their side effect and risk profiles. Further research on male contraceptives is needed to determine their acceptability and safety, particularly for adolescent males.

QUESTIONS

1. You are seeing an 18-year-old female for contraceptive management. She is taking Depo-Provera, but she has missed the time frame for her scheduled injections several times. She has gained 10 pounds and continues to have intermittent breakthrough bleeding after a year of taking Depo-Provera. You discuss the possibility of long-acting reversible contraception, but she is not interested. She has been researching alternative contraceptive options online and asks about the potential use of subcutaneous medroxyprogesterone acetate (DMPA-SC). Which of the following is a potential advantage of using DMPA-SC for this patient?
   A. Less weight gain
   B. Menstrual suppression
   C. Ease of administration
   D. Similar administration schedule as Depo-Provera
2. You are working with a third-year medical student in your clinic. The student observes a clinical encounter with a 19-year-old female requesting removal of the copper intrauterine device (IUD) because of worsening

menstrual cramps. After this encounter, the student asks if newer versions of copper IUDs cause less discomfort. Which of the following features of the IUDs in development helps reduce discomfort?
A. Flexible memory frame
B. Smaller inserter
C. Reduced copper dosage

3. You are planning to give a lecture on future developments in male contraception, which includes alternatives to vasectomies, such as reversible inhibition of sperm under guidance (RISUG) and Vasalgel. Which of the following best describes the function of RISUG and Vasalgel for pregnancy prevention?
A. Affect sperm function
B. Block sperm transport
C. Inhibit spermatogenesis

(See pages 204-205 for answers.)

References

1. Adolescent pregnancy and its outcomes across countries. Guttmacher Institute. https://www.guttmacher.org/fact-sheet/adolescent-pregnancy-and-its-outcomes-across-countries. August 2015. Accessed May 20, 2018
2. Lindberg LD, Santelli J, Desai S. Understanding the decline in adolescent fertility in the United States, 2007-2012. *J Adolesc Health*. 2016;59:577-583
3. American Academy of Pediatrics Committee on Adolescence. Contraception for adolescents. *Pediatrics*. 2014;134:e1244-e1256
4. ACOG Committee Opinion No. 735: Adolescents and long-acting reversible contraception: implants and intrauterine devices. *Obstet Gynecol*. 2018;131:e130-e139
5. Contraceptive use. Centers for Disease Control and Prevention. https://www.cdc.gov/nchs/fastats/contraceptive.htm. Updated July 15, 2016. Accessed June 12, 2018
6. United Nations, Department of Economic and Social Affairs, Population Division. *World Family Planning 2017–Highlights* (ST/ESA/SER.A/414). New York: United Nations; 2017
7. Buhling KJ, Zite N, Lotke P, Black K. Worldwide use of intrauterine contraception: a review. *Contraception*. 2014;89:162-173
8. Thompson K. A brief history of birth control in the U.S. https://www.ourbodiesourselves.org/book-excerpts/health-article/a-brief-history-of-birth-control/. December 14, 2013. Accessed on July 15, 2018
9. Hubacher D. The checkered history and bright future of intrauterine contraception in the United States. *Perspect Reprod Sex Health*. 2002;34:98-103
10. Keith BM. Home-based administration of depo-subQ provera 104 in the Uniject injection system: a literature review. Seattle, WA: Program for Appropriate Technology in Health (PATH); 2011
11. Sayana Press (DMPA-SC in Uniject) Product and Project Summary. Program for Appropriate Technology in Health (PATH). https://path.azureedge.net/media/documents/RH_sp_project_summary.pdf. January 2017. Accessed May 20, 2018
12. Cover J, Namagembe A, Tumusiime J, Lim J, Drake JK, Mbonye AK. A prospective cohort study of the feasibility and acceptability of depot medroxyprogesterone acetate administered subcutaneously through self-injection. *Contraception*. 2017;95:306-311

13. Cover J, Lim J, Namagembe A, Tumusiime J, Kidwell Drake J, Muntifering Cox C. Acceptability of contraceptive self-injection with DMPA-SC among adolescents in Gulu District, Uganda. *Int Perspect Sex Reprod Health.* 2017;43:153-162
14. Reproductive Health Supplies Coalition. Caucus on New and Underused Reproductive Health Technologies. Product Brief: Female Condom. https://www.rhsupplies.org/fileadmin/uploads/rhsc/Working_Groups/New_Underused_RH_Technologies_Caucus/Documents/Technical_Briefs/rhsc-brief-female-condom_A4.pdf. Updated May 2013. Accessed November 26, 2018
15. Microchips technology. Microchips Biotech. http://microchipsbiotech.com/technology.php. Accessed June 12, 2018
16. Kinkead G. A contraceptive implant with remote control. https://www.technologyreview.com/s/528121/a-contraceptive-implant-with-remote-control/. Published July 4, 2014. Accessed June 12, 2018
17. Farra R, Sheppard N, McCabe L, et al. First-in-human testing of a wirelessly controlled drug delivery microchip. *Sci Transl Med.* 2012;4:122ra21
18. Evaluation of Efficacy, Safety, and Tolerability of VeraCept IUD. https://clinicaltrials.gov/ct2/show/study/NCT03633799#locn. Accessed on November 22, 2018
19. Reeves M, Hathaway M, Canela Oleaga JM, Katz BH, Tal MG. A randomized single-blinded trial of Veracept, a novel nitinol low-dose copper intrauterine contraceptive compared with a copper T380S intrauterine contraceptive. Abstract Oral Presentation. American College of Obstetricians and Gynecologists Annual Clinical and Scientific Meeting. San Francisco, CA. May 2015
20. Evaluation of the Efficacy and Safety of LevoCept. https://clinicaltrials.gov/ct2/show/study/NCT02882191. Accessed November 22, 2018
21. The next generation IUD: IUB SCu300. OCON Medicall. https://www.oconmed.com/en/contraception/intrauterine-ball-iub/. Accessed June 12, 2018
22. Wiebe E, Trussell J. Discontinuation rates and acceptability during 1 year of using the intrauterine ball (the SCU380A). *Contraception.* 2016;93:364-366
23. Li Y, Zhang SM, Chen F, et al. A multi-center randomized controlled trial of intrauterine use in Chinese women. *Zhonghua Yi Xue Za Zhi.* 2011;91:3172-3175
24. FDA approves new vaginal ring for one year of birth control. US Food and Drug Administration. https://www.fda.gov/NewsEvents/Newsroom/PressAnnouncements/ucm616541.htm. Published August 10, 2018. Accessed August 14, 2018
25. Birth control on the horizon: 2016 edition. Bedsider. https://www.bedsider.org/features/911-birth-control-on-the-horizon-2016-edition. July 2016. Accessed May 20, 2018
26. Baeten JM, Palanee-Phillips T, Brown ER, et al. Use of a vaginal ring containing dapivirine for HIV-1 prevention in women. *N Engl J Med.* 2016;375:2121-2132
27. Kanakis G, Goulis D. Male contraception: a clinically oriented review. *Hormones.* 2015;14:589-614
28. Khourdaji I, Zillioux J, Eisenfrats I, Foley D, Smith R. The future of male contraception: a fertile ground. *Transl Androl Urol.* 2018;7:S220-S235
29. Male Contraceptives Initiative. Contraceptives in active development. https://www.malecontraceptive.org/prospective/. Accessed November 26, 2018
30. Nya-Ngatchou JJ, Amory JK. New approaches to male non-hormonal contraception. *Contraception.* 2013;87:296-299

Adolesc Med 030 (2019) 196–205

Answers to Questions

Contraceptive Use by US Adolescents: Where Are We Now? **Page 1**

1. *Answer:* B. According to data from the CDC, there was no statistically significant change in condom or IUD use reported by 15- to 19-year-olds since 2006.

2. *Answer:* A. The two most important national surveys providing information on teen sexual behavior and contraceptive use are the Youth Risk Behavior Surveillance System and National Survey of Family Growth. The YRBSS is conducted every two years and provides nationally representative data on students in grades 9-12. The National Survey of Family Growth is a nationally representative sample of reproductive age persons. In 2015, the age range of participants in the NSFG was changed to encompass those ages 15-49 years. In 2006, the NSFG methodology changed from periodic data collection to continuous collection.

3. *Answer:* C. It is important for adolescents to be aware of the range of contraceptive options and their attributes, including effectiveness. For some adolescents, potential side effects of a method may outweigh potential benefits, including risk of method failure. Identifying the attributes of a method most important to the individual adolescent can help tailor contraceptive counseling.

Adolescent Pregnancy Prevention: Application of CDC Evidence-Based Contraception Guidance **Page 10**

1. *Answer:* B. According to the US MEC's numeric scheme, a contraceptive method classified as a category 2 for a specific medical condition indicates that the advantages of using the contraceptive method generally outweigh the theoretical or proven risks.

2. *Answer:* C. The adolescent can have the implant placed today. She does not need a pregnancy test since she has no signs or symptoms of pregnancy and meets at least one criterion from US Selected Practice Recommenda-

tions for Contraceptive Use (US SPR) guidance on how to be reasonably certain that a woman is not pregnant (ie, she is no more than 7 days after the start of normal menses). She does not need to abstain from sex or use backup contraception for the next 7 days given the timing of her last menses. She does not meet age criteria for cervical cytology screening, and generally, this testing does not contribute substantially to safe and effective use of the implant.

3. *Answer:* A. The US SPR provides guidance on the examinations and tests needed before initiation of specific contraceptive methods for women presumed to be healthy. For combined hormonal methods, including COCs, blood pressure should be measured before initiation. The adolescent does not meet age criteria for cervical cytology screening and does not need to have a clinical breast examination, bimanual examination, or hemoglobin test, since these tests do not contribute substantially to safe and effective use of COCs. However, these examinations and tests might be appropriate for diagnosing or assessing suspected medical conditions.

4. *Answer:* E. Emergency contraception provides protection against pregnancy up to 120 hours after intercourse that occurs without any contraception or with a contraceptive failure (eg, broken condom). The adolescent can safely use all the emergency contraception options listed (ie, Cu-IUD, ulipristal acetate emergency contraceptive pills, levonorgestrel emergency contraceptive pills, and combination estrogen/progestin pills). Her choice of which emergency contraception option to use will likely depend on access and her plans to initiate regular contraception after use of emergency contraception.

5. *Answer:* A. If the adolescent chooses to use levonorgestrel emergency contraceptive pills, she can start the vaginal ring immediately. If the adolescent chooses to use ulipristal acetate emergency contraceptive pills, she should start the vaginal ring no sooner than 5 days after use of the pills. This is because ulipristial acetate is an antiprogestin and may interact with hormonal contraception and decrease the effectiveness of the ulipristal acetate pills. The adolescent does not need to wait until her next menses or after a negative pregnancy test to initiate the vaginal ring.

6. *Answer*: B. The adolescent can start the LNG-IUD today. She also can be screened for STIs today according to STI screening guidelines, but LNG-IUD placement should not be delayed. She does not need to be treated presumptively for chlamydial and gonococcal infection. If she tests positive for either infection, she can be treated without removing the IUD.

Incorporating the Adolescent in Individualized and Effective Contraceptive Counseling **Page 24**

1. *Answer:* D. All 3 patient priorities deserve exploring at the contraceptive counseling visit. Choice A addresses a potential need for a highly confidential method if her family would disapprove of birth control. Choice B is an important topic to address with any female patient of reproductive age. It can be helpful for the patient to start thinking ahead in her life plan and is helpful for the clinician to be able to offer timeline-appropriate birth control methods. Finally, Choice C may not seem like a priority at a contraceptive counseling visit, however, as it was expressed as "the patient's concerns about her mental health", it becomes a priority for the visit because it is *her* priority. This may lead to discussion and screening for depression, or it may simply be a concern she has for birth control increasing her emotional lability that she heard was possible. Either way, if the patient brings up a concern or question, then it is a priority for the visit. Enquiring about safety and future family planning are less obvious yet practical priorities that might make a difference to the patient in her decision.

2. *Answer:* B. Choice B is the only clinician response that attempts to evoke the patient's priorities. Asking a patient for reasons she favors condoms may reveal that she likes *in the moment* spontaneity. If this is her biggest priority about birth control, then with permission, the clinician could suggest other options that could also offer her spontaneity, while continuing to congratulate the patient on condom use to prevent infections. Discussing her dislikes about condoms may help the patient come to some new conclusions about her priorities and interest in other forms of birth control. Choices A and C reflect a judgmental provider. Both A and C may at first seem like a reflection of the patient's behavior, however, they may inadvertently assign guilt to her choice of condoms and display an obvious provider preference of what she should be using. In choice D, the clinician assumes that the patient has enough condoms and ends the conversation. While there could be many reasons that condoms might not work well for this patient every time, access to condoms is not likely the reason.

3. *Answer:* B. The only medically contraindicated choice is an estrogen containing-method such as the vaginal ring. The patient identifies her priorities as wanting to avoid any possible weight gain and not wanting anyone to know she's using birth control. The method of choice that would be least likely to change her periods or cause amenorrhea while at the same time being undetectable by a sexual partner would be the Copper IUD (B). The hormonal IUD could possibly be an option as well, as not all patients experience amenorrhea. Using a smaller hormonal IUD such as Kyleena

or Skyla could allow the patient to continue getting periods while providing excellent contraception. For confidentiality, strings on the IUD can be cut shorter to avoid partner detection. In this scenario, it would be recommended to also assess the patient for domestic violence and safety.

New Approaches for Pregnancy Prevention: Getting Males Involved With Both Male- and Female-Dependent Methods of Contraception Page 34

1. *Answer:* B. This patient's girlfriend is reluctant to discuss any type of contraception with her healthcare practitioner because she is concerned that her parents will find out that she is sexually active. While many adolescents can obtain contraception from their practitioner through confidential services, many adolescent girls may not do so because of concern that someone, including their parents, will find out. Given these concerns, it is unlikely that this patient's girlfriend would be willing to obtain emergency contraception including a copper IUD from her practitioner. This method would also not be ideal for her given she has a history of heavy and painful periods. Obtaining ella via the online consultation is a possibility but the patient's girlfriend would need to have it delivered to a place outside of her home if she does not want her parents to find out. Plan B would be the easiest to access for the patient and his girlfriend, its use would be more private so that patient's girlfriend would feel more comfortable using it, and would still be effective given only 2 days have passed since the condom slippage incident. It also allows the male in this situation to take a more active role in pregnancy prevention and to be supportive of his partner by allowing him to purchase Plan B if patient's girlfriend desires to use it. However, there could still be some challenges with obtaining Plan B including the cost to pay for it out of pocket.

2. *Answer:* D. While the father appears to have his son's best interests in mind in this scenario, it would be inappropriate to break confidentiality and tell the patient's father about the patient's sexual practices. Answer A is therefore incorrect. Answer B reminds the father that you will provide confidential services to his son which is important in any adolescent health visit. Answer C is also correct given that when adolescents discuss sex, condoms, and contraception with their parents they are more likely to practice safe sex given that these discussions may increase their ability to negotiate condoms and contraception with their partners. It is also important to try to teach this father some key points about condoms and contraception as some fathers may have limited knowledge about these topics.

3. *Answer:* C. All of the statements about condoms are true except that they are not the most effective male-dependent form of contraception. Vasectomy is the most effective form of male-dependent contraception. As a

reminder, oil-based lubricants should not be used with latex condoms given that they increase the risk that they will break, but water- or silicone-based lubricants can be used.

4. *Answer:* F. Answers A, B, D, and E incorporate motivational interviewing into the discussion with the patient and give the patient more control over what he wishes to learn about and do. Using this approach would allow the practitioner to establish better rapport with the patient in this situation. Answer C is incorrect because it is very judgmental and may cause the patient to become distant and to resist receiving some of the advice or guidance that you could provide.

5. *Answer:* E. A sexual health curriculum focusing on abstinence or one that teaches males about only condoms and females only about contraception are not ideal for providing adolescents with the most knowledge to reduce their risk of being involved in an unintended pregnancy or of acquiring an STI. Discussing condoms and contraception with all students regardless of their sex and providing students with condoms and contraception at their school would be more helpful in this regard.

Condoms On and Off: A Review of Prophylactic Barrier Use and Youth Sexual Well-Being **Page 45**

1. *Answer:* D. Rates of use of penis-covering barriers during penis–vulva/vagina sex are quite high for first partnered experiences: up to 80% or more, depending on the data source.

2. *Answer:* A. Penis size is associated with breakage of penis-covering barriers, especially with penis–anus/rectum sex.

3. *Answer:* C. Vulvar/vaginal/pelvic pain associated with penis–vulva/vagina sex is common, perhaps more so with penis-covering barriers.

The Contraceptive Ring, Patch, and Pills: An Update **Page 60**

1. *Answer:* C. Begin with the most likely causes and least invasive intervention. The most likely cause is that she is taking it on an empty stomach or during the day.

2. *Answer:* B. After 2 months, it's time to intervene. Start with the least invasive/disruptive treatment. Ibuprofen generally will decrease bleeding by 30%.

3. *Answer:* C. Drosperinone has the least androgenic effect, norgestimate has an intermediate androgenic effect, and levonorgestrel has the most androgenic effect of the 3 progestins listed.

4. *Answer:* A. Levonorgestrel has the most androgenic effect, norgestimate has an intermediate androgenic effect, while drosperinone has the least androgenic effect of the 3 progestins listed.

5. *Answer:* C. In women of bone accrual age (15-30 years of age), 30 mcg of ethinyl estradiol is the minimum dose of estrogen needed to maintain good bone health.

Depo-Provera: Is It Still a Good Option for Adolescents? Page 82

1. *Answer:* B. Early weight gain, defined as >5% increase over baseline at 6 months of use, is currently the best predictor of continued excessive weight gain on DMPA. Adolescents who have gained ≤5% of baseline weight at 6 months can be reassured that they are unlikely to experience excessive weight gain on this method. These patients should continue to have their weight monitored and receive routine diet and exercise counseling. Among adolescents who do experience early weight gain, risks and benefits of continued DMPA use should be weighed carefully, including risk of unintended pregnancy with method discontinuation.

2. *Answer:* A. It is important to first obtain a detailed description of the bleeding pattern and to distinguish bleeding that is bothersome to the adolescent from that which is tolerable or insignificant. Only bothersome bleeding requires treatment. Current evidence does not support that either DMPA dose or frequency of injections affects menstrual pattern. As this patient had recent negative STI screens and denies sexual activity since last STI screening, her irregular bleeding is less likely related to an STI at this time.

3. *Answer:* C. Current clinical guidelines recommend that health care professionals continue to prescribe DMPA to adolescents with full discussion of risks and benefits and not limit DMPA use to 2 years. There is no indication for BMD monitoring in an otherwise healthy adolescent using DMPA. Bone mineral density assessment may be considered in adolescents with other risk factors for low BMD. Per the U.S. Medical Eligibility Criteria for Contraceptive Use, adolescence is a category 2 condition in which the advantages of DMPA use generally outweigh the risks in this age group.

Intrauterine Devices for Adolescents: Guidance for Clinicians **Page 102**

1. *Answer:* B. There is no age that is a contraindication to IUD use. Clinicians should ensure that a patient has achieved menarche and is cognitively mature enough to engage meaningfully in the informed consent process.

2. *Answer:* D. Oral contraceptive pills have typical use failure rates of 9% while IUD typical use failure rates are <1%. There is no minimum duration for which an IUD must be left in place prior to removal. Most IUD users have less menstrual bleeding 1 year after insertion than at baseline.

3. *Answer:* C. IUD expulsion rates range from 3% to 20% and can occur even with proper insertion. The copper IUD is approved by the FDA for emergency contraception for up to 5 days after unprotected sexual intercourse, and lidocaine is effective in reducing pain associated with IUD insertion via paracervical block or topical gel.

A "Call To Arms": Using the Contraceptive Implant to Reduce Unplanned Adolescent Pregnancy **Page 118**

1. *Answer:* A. This patient has a contraindication to estrogen-containing methods of contraception due to a history of deep venous thrombosis, a desire for the most effective contraception, and desires pregnancy in 2-3 years; therefore, the etonogestrel implant is the best option for the patient in this scenario.

2. *Answer:* D. In a patient with a normal hemoglobin, irregular bleeding pattern, and no suspicion for a sexually transmitted infection, the first step to manage breakthrough bleeding would be naproxen 500 mg twice daily for 5 days.

3. *Answer:* C. For a patient who has estrogen contraindication of migraine with aura, a contraindication to intrauterine device placement because of pelvic inflammatory disease, and is desiring the most effect contraception the best choice would be the etonogestrel implant. Of the answers provided, the only correct answer is that ovulation resumes within 10 to 14 days after discontinuation.

When "Plan A" Fails: Emergency Contraception **Page 134**

1. *Answer:* C. For maximum efficacy between 72 to 120 hours postcoitus, ulipristal acetate and the copper IUD are the best options for EC. However, when reviewing all considerations in this case, the best option for this patient is the copper IUD, the only method not affected by BMI.

2. *Answer:* E. For an individual considering EC in advance, many options are available. Although routine preventive contraception methods are encouraged, it is important to be aware of all available options. Advanced provision of EC is recommended by organizations such as the American Academy of Pediatrics, American College of Obstetricians and Gynecologists, Society for Adolescent Health and Medicine, and American Academy of Family Physicians. All of the answers are appropriate if EC is necessary, despite barriers that might affect how easy they are to obtain.

3. *Answer:* D. While teaching this individual preventive methods (choice E) for the future is important, it will not address the events of the previous night. Choice B is also encouraged, but it is an extra obstacle that might delay a time-sensitive medication. Choice C should be performed, but it will not affect the possibility of preventing a pregnancy, and it is too soon to test for STIs from this exposure.

Implementation of LARC Methods Into Pediatric Practice **Page 150**

1. *Answer:* C. Irregular bleeding occurs commonly after IUD placement. If there is no other underlying problem (eg, STI or displacement), consider short-term treatment with NSAIDs or hormonal treatment with oral contraceptives or estrogen.

2. *Answer:* C. In a recent Cochrane review, lidocaine 2% gel had no effect on pain during IUD insertion or tenaculum placement. Misoprostol was associated with higher pain scores and more cramping than placebo groups. Pain with IUD insertion was less with tramadol versus naproxen; however, in the same trial, pain was less with naproxen compared to placebo.

3. *Answer:* B. If an implant is not palpable at a follow-up visit, pregnancy should be excluded, and backup contraception provided until the presence of the implant is confirmed.

Special Cases: Case-Based Contraception Scenarios **Page 161**

1. *Answer:* B. Nexplanon is a radiopaque rod and therefore a radiograph should be sufficient in locating the implant in the arm. It is the simplest and quickest type of radiologic study to obtain.

2. *Answer:* C. The case should prompt a clinician to assess the position of the IUD. Visualization of IUD strings during a pelvic examination in the office is a simple procedure that could provide information on the location of the IUD. If the strings are not visualized then further steps such as urine pregnancy test and ultrasound are required.

3. *Answer:* E. Implants have not been studied for the treatment of heavy or prolonged uterine bleeding, and copper IUDs cause an increase in the amount of uterine bleeding. Both combined hormonal contraceptive pills and levonorgestrel IUDs have been shown to reduce the amount of uterine bleeding in women with von Willebrand disease.

Policy Foundations Supporting Adolescent Access to Contraceptive Care **Page 174**

1. *Answer:* B. Regarding sexual and reproductive health care, many states explicitly permit all or some minors to obtain contraceptive, prenatal, and STI services without parental involvement. If a state or jurisdiction does not have specific provisions for minors' consent for contraception services, then these services fall under the states' general statutes for minors' consent for medical care. When minors obtain care under Title X or Medicaid funding, then these programs guarantee consent for contraception.

2. *Answer:* C. With few exceptions, the Affordable Care Act mandates insurance coverage of all FDA-approved contraception services without co-payment; however, the ability to request confidential communications vary by state. There are no federal confidentiality protections with the exception of Title X and Medicaid funded services.

3. *Answer:* B. Several states have (California, Oregon) or passed (Maryland, Illinois) laws allowing pharmacy access to hormonal contraception. Nationally, emergency contraception is available over the counter without a prescription without an age restriction for levonorgestrel products only. Ulipristal EC requires a prescription.

New Contraceptive Developments on the Horizon **Page 187**

1. *Answer:* C. This patient is having difficulty with coming in for scheduled Depo-Provera injections. DMPA-SC could potentially be advantageous for this patient since it can be self-administered, which would eliminate access barriers that the patient may have to get to her appointments. DMPA-SC has similar side effects as Depo-Provera, including weight gain and irregular bleeding patterns. Therefore, choice A and B are not correct. DMPA-SC does have the same dosing schedule as Depo-Provera, however, the patient missed several scheduled Depo-Provera injections. Therefore, choice D is not a potential advantage for this patient.

2. *Answer:* A. The flexible memory frame changes shape in relation to the uterus to help reduce discomfort. Research showed that participants using the IUD composed of the flexible memory frame had lower discontinuation rates compared to the current copper IUD available in the United States. Some of the newer IUDs have a smaller inserter, which would elicit less pain only on insertion. The copper dosage does not relate to the level of pain.

3. *Answer:* B. Reversible inhibition of sperm under guidance (RISUG) and Vasalgel both function by blocking sperm transport. Although side effects of these procedures affect sperm function, this is not the intended mechanism of action.

Adolesc Med 030 (2019) 207–215

Note: Page numbers of articles are in **boldface** type. Page references followed by "*f*" and "*t*" denote figures and tables, respectively.

A

B

C

D

Q

R

S

T

U